Psychosurgery

Psychosurgery

DAMAGING THE BRAIN
TO SAVE THE MIND

Joann Ellison Rodgers

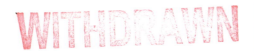

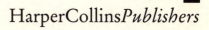

HarperCollins*Publishers*

HarperCollins books may be purchased for educational, business, or sales promotional use. For information, please call or write: Special Markets Department, HarperCollins Publishers, Inc., 10 East 53rd Street, New York, NY 10022. Telephone: (212) 207-7528; Fax: (212) 207-7222.

FIRST EDITION

Designed by Cassandra Pappas

Library of Congress Cataloging-in-Publication Data

Rodgers, Joann Ellison.
    Psychosurgery : damaging the brain to save the mind / Joann Ellison Rodgers.—1st ed.
        p.   cm.
    Includes bibliographical references and index.
    ISBN 0-06-016405-0 (cloth)
    1. Psychosurgery. I. Title.
    [DNLM: 1. Psychosurgery.   WL 370 R691p]
    RD594.R63 1992
    617.4′81—dc20
    DNLM/DLC
    for Library of Congress   91-50436

92 93 94 95 96 ❖/RRD 10 9 8 7 6 5 4 3 2 1

For my parents, Dorothy Hirschhorn Ellison and Max Ellison

One must have a good memory to be able to keep the promises one makes.

—Friedrich Wilhelm Nietzsche, *Human, All Too Human*

Contents

FOREWORD

Philosophers tell us that the horizon of knowledge is always out of reach. How far out of reach is the practical question and the source of all dilemmas having to do with treating the sick. Do doctors wait until they really know—or know more—before they try this or that treatment? If they wait, will it mean more suffering for a patient? Is suffering tolerable if there are means of relieving it? Are some risks ever worth taking? Are some ever not?

The treatment dilemma posed by psychosurgery—surgery to treat psychiatric disorders—is this: experts know something about mental illness and about operations that can help some patients, but they don't know enough to completely assure patients, families, or the rest of us that surgery is the best or proper course, that it is ever worth the risk.

Perhaps they never can know enough. Driving the demand for, and use of, psychosurgery is the belief—some call it the pretension—that the human brain can understand and repair its own mind; and more, that scientists will come to understand the mind and brain better by studying them the way they study them now: anatomically, biochemically, and empirically, by analyzing and observing their parts and the things they do.

But is that belief reasonable or true? Might there be a better way of approaching the horizon of the mind, of seeing it better? Is there a different pair of binoculars with a different kind of focus that scientists have not yet even conjured in minds bent to the way science has been done—and applied—for the past 100 years?

It is pretentious to assume our scientists—or our philosophers for that matter—can sort out the intricate connections among mind, brain, and behavior. And I believe there probably is a better pair of binoculars. But should doctors wait until they find all—or more—or better—answers and paths to knowledge before they act to relieve suffering? No.

With rare exceptions, the authorities whose ideas are described in these pages are thoughtful about all of this. They wanted readers of this book to know that they worry a lot about what they don't know and what may never be known. But even the least philosophical of them suspects that science cannot resolve dilemmas generated by the nature, origins, and limits of human knowledge. Said one: "We are always actors asked to perform with unfinished scripts, before a full house, and we fear a missed cue far more than a missing line."

So far as this observer can tell, the history of medicine and psychiatry affirms their view that the way out of the therapeutic dilemma is to grab the proverbial bull by both horns (thereby avoiding a fatal wound from either side) and to steer the course as best they can.

Psychosurgery, drugs, electroconvulsive therapy, and all physical means ever devised to treat mental illness and related disorders are profoundly risky. But they are, for now, for our time, the best available. The challenge is to use them selectively and humanely, to accept that whatever is done puts people in harm's way, and to acknowledge and nurture the bravery among the treaters and the treated who must ride the bull.

ACKNOWLEDGMENTS

First among the many who supported this work is Pamela Jane Gray Sherman, whose research skills jump started the project. At the Johns Hopkins Medical Institutions, the home of biological psychiatry, thanks go to the Welch Medical Library staff; to Bernice Coles, my assistant in the Office of Public Affairs; and to Guy McKhann, Gert Brieger, Donlin Long, John Freeman, Peter Fox, Haring Nauta, Bob Fisher, Paul McHugh, Sol Snyder, and other members of the medical school faculty for stretching my reach around an ever-expanding subject.

More than 40 psychiatrists, neurologists, neurosurgeons, ethicists, medical historians, social scientists, and lawyers lent their time, ideas, and enthusiasm to the work. Most are quoted in the text, but special mentions are owed to Michael Shapiro, J.D., of the University of Southern California School of Law; Louis Jolyn West, M.D., of the University of California at Los Angeles Medical Center's Neuropsychiatric Institute; H. Thomas Ballantine, M.D., of Massachusetts General Hospital and Harvard University School of Medicine; Robert A. Burt, J.D., of Yale University School of Law; Andrew Scull, Ph.D., of the University of California, San Diego; Desmond Kelly, M.D., of the Priory Hospital in London; Paul Bridges, M.D., of the Geoffrey Knight National Unit for Affective Disorders at Guy's Hospital in London; and

Geoffrey Cureton Knight, M.D., neurosurgical consultant (retired), London.

Larry Ashmead at HarperCollins, who proposed the book, has my gratitude for a chance in his "house." So, too, does my agent and friend Elaine Markson.

To my sons, Adam and Jared, thank you for so much love, support, and late-night counsel, offered always amid demanding commitments of your own. And to Robert Henry Nath: Thank you for making time for us when I needed it most.

For friends and strangers who shared their stories and helped me understand the devastation that mental illness visits on families, no words can settle the debt; it remains. And to the mentally ill men and women whose lives are documentaries of almost unspeakable woe, you have my everlasting respect for your courage.

JOANN ELLISON RODGERS
Baltimore, Maryland

INTRODUCTION

Why now, almost 30 years after psychiatrists and neurosurgeons abandoned lobotomies, is there a new book about psychosurgery? Why now, so long after the counterculture successfully and universally made lobotomy a metaphor for therapeutic barbarism and equated any kind of brain surgery for psychiatric illness with malevolent government mind control of dissidents and criminals, armies of zombies, suppression of civil rights, and immoral, abusive medical care? Why now, when psychosurgery on children, prisoners, involuntary or legally incompetent patients is banned in all federally supported hospitals? Why now, when doctors have a drugstore full of tranquilizers and antidepressants?

The answer is that strong ideas survive, even if they sometimes led to bad acts and disillusionment and especially if they sometimes led to good acts and benefits. The idea of treating certain mental conditions permanently, effectively, and safely with surgical means is one of those ideas. It's an idea that has come, gone, and is here again. Or, more accurately, is here still.

This will come as a surprise to many, even to many psychiatrists. It was certainly a surprise to me. I had paid no attention whatever to the subject of psychiatric brain surgery since 1978, when one of my assignments as national science correspondent for the Hearst newspapers was to write a story on a report issued by the National Commission for the Protection of Human Subjects of

Biomedical and Behavioral Research. Among other things, the report concluded that psychosurgery had a deservedly bad reputation for wretched excess, but also some documented successes; that it was not the unmitigated horror its critics labeled it; that with strict regulations and safeguards psychosurgery was acceptable for certain cases; and that more research and good record keeping were needed.

To background my article, I spent a few hours in the newspaper "morgue," alternately buoyed by the hope psychosurgery gave to many and repelled by the gruesome stories of "ice-pick" prefrontal lobotomies. In the end, I concluded that the commission's findings and the guidelines it recommended for doing psychosurgery were essentially moot; the procedures and those who embraced them were all but gone from the scene or at least underground by then. My scientific sources agreed; psychosurgery was a dead issue and no good would come of spending any more time and energy on the topic. In fact, I spent some of the next ten years writing stories about the pharmacologic and psychiatric advances that had buried it.

Thus, late in 1988, I was puzzled by the invitation to write a book about psychosurgery. What was there to report?

As it turned out, there was a great deal. After a few months of phone inquiries and library research, I had an outline that would take two years to fill in. I had evidence that psychosurgery—albeit under new names, more refined and more selective—was still very much around; it had, actually, never completely gone away.

Neurosurgeons and psychiatrists at prestigious institutions were calling—in soft, but nevertheless clear voices—for new research in mind and mood-altering surgery, their interest fed by the side effects and failures of talk therapies and long-term drug use in the sickest mental patients.

Moreover, I discovered that the hard lessons of the past had not so much been passed on as passed over; there were still those willing, even eager, to abuse the power of psychiatry and neurosurgery to achieve their personal visions of social order. The psychiatric community, the courts, watchdog associations, and regulatory agencies never came to grips with how to weigh the risks and benefits for patients. And the newer techniques available to brain surgeons potentially made abuse even easier for modern operators than an unregulated, unfettered free hand had made it for early psychosurgeons. As historian David Shutts wrote in his 1982 book on lobotomies, "the specter of creating submissive zombies loomed larger as contemporary stereotactic surgeons were better able to pinpoint the destruction of specific areas of the brain, particularly the amygdala nucleus in the temporal lobe, which is believed to be involved in eliciting violent behavior." (A 1990 mystery/adventure by novelist Caryl Rivers, *Indecent Behaviors*, has brought that specter home for a generation that never heard of Ken Kesey's Randle McMurphy in *One Flew Over the Cuckoo's Nest*.)

So there is new promise and new peril to report. Although the numbers of procedures performed have plunged since the heyday of psychosurgery (50,000 estimated in the United States alone between 1936 and 1960), there are still at least 200 to 300 openly declared psychosurgeries being performed each year by a few dozen surgeons here and abroad. Reports are trickling in of more operations being done in South America and the developing world. And if operations that affect the "psyche" but disclaim changes in mood and behavior as primary goals are counted, the total is certainly higher and growing.

As uncomfortable as it seemed to me to jump into a subject that had no popular champion, no constituency even remotely classy, and no official voice, so also was it irresistible. Every American family, according to the National Institute of Mental Health, has at least one mentally ill member and a right to know about *every* treatment option open to patients. For some of the millions worldwide languishing in institutions, on the streets, or at home with intractable and disabling mental illness, surgery could be a threat but could also be a benefit that is systematically and unfairly denied them by disinterest, fear, and heavy political opposition.

So what began as an invitation to popularize a bleak chapter in psychiatry's past became a summons to a very different task. My out-of-date biases fell before current information. Newly gathered facts drove the story in surprising directions. Surgeons no longer destroy large amounts of brain tissue in futile efforts to "cure" schizophrenia and neurosis. Instead, they take pinpoint aim at millimeter-long clusters of cells to stop suicidal depression, disabling obsessive-compulsive disorder, crippling anxiety, and uncontrollable rage and aggression that keep sick people in locked wards. They go after destructive behavior that accompanies organic diseases of the body and brain.

Dams of silence and shame are crumbling. In Britain, psychiatrists John Bartlett, Paul Bridges, and Desmond Kelly, contemporary advocates of psychosurgery, acknowledge the excesses of the past, but call firmly, in a recent publication, for "a reappraisal of the therapeutic possibilities of the modern refined operations." An operation called a stereotactic subcaudate tractotomy, developed by their colleague, Geoffrey Knight, has been performed on more than 1,200 patients in Britain in recent years, with the blessing of Britain's Mental Health Act Commission. Said Bridges in a 1988 article in *The Journal of Neurosurgery*, "psychosurgery retains a place in the treatment of a small, highly selected group of patients."

In the United States, the chief of neurosurgery at the Johns Hopkins Medical Institutions, Donlin Long, told me that "abandonment of psychosurgery in concept and practice has been of tremendous detriment to patients. We forget," he continued, "that even with the worst of the past's excesses, lobotomies helped some. Just think what we might do now with more knowledge and less destructive techniques such as electrostimulation of brain tissue."

These are not words that describe disinterest or a dead issue.

On the other hand, I also learned that fear of legal, political, and regulatory repercussions conspire still to keep information about new developments so low profile as to be virtually invisible to the public and to journalists who report to the public on health and medicine. For example, some of the psychiatrists and surgeons who made headlines calling for an open mind about psychosurgery in the 1970s would not respond to repeated requests for interviews. Others sat for interviews but dove for cover behind *mea culpas*. One neurologist at a prestigious East Coast medical center made anonymity for himself and his hospital the price of cooperation and access to information. (Interestingly, neither his patient nor his patient's family felt that way.)

Before agreeing to see me, Britain's Paul Bridges sternly lectured me by letter to avoid "slipping into vituperation that tends to afflict non-psychiatrists when dealing with this subject.... It has been done so many times before—why bother?" And without exception, every surgeon and psychiatrist I interviewed requested that the word *psychosurgery* be expunged from the text in favor of such phrases as "brain surgery to treat psychiatric diagnoses" or "functional neurosurgery." In the summer of 1990, in an editorial in the *Journal of Neuropsychiatry*, the editors suggested yet another substitute phrase: "NRI" for "neurosurgical and related interventions" for the treatment of patients with psychiatric disorders. (Readers please note: I'm sympathetic, but in the interests of brevity and style, I'll use a variety of phrases—including *psychosurgery*—throughout the book.)

In the 1990s, dubbed the "Decade of the Brain" by the National Academy of Sciences, a few advocates of the mentally ill and some doctors are responding positively to suggestions for new research on the subject. Hospitals are convening special internal review panels to consider requests for psychosurgery. And young surgeons, teamed with psychiatrists, are learning to put advanced neurosurgical skills in service to psychiatric patients.

What else is there to report? The critics. For some, the abuses of the past remain open sores on the national conscience. Washington psychiatrist Peter Breggin, among others, passionately continues to brand as evil anyone interested in psychosurgery and to link any renewed efforts to ulterior political motives or Frankenstein-style science. Others dismiss the whole idea as just plain goofy and based on oversimplified views of human behavior and emotional chaos. Pseudoreligious groups, like the Scientologists, label psychosurgery and all physical ("somatic") treatment of mental illness as assassination attempts on the mind.

At the very least, it seemed to me that the facts about psychosurgery, like the illnesses it targets, were too complicated to ignore or gloss over and were, therefore, worth examining. However much some gag at the thought, psychosurgery had honest purpose and successes—and is still having them. "No one who has not witnessed the utter despair and misery of the chronically mentally ill can truly appreciate why members of the medical community and mental health professionals embraced psychosurgery and still do," Boston neurosurgeon Tom Ballantine told me. Now retired from the operating room, Ballantine heads a panel at Massachusetts General Hospital that reviews requests for modified psychosurgical procedures on mentally ill patients there. "I am very much their advocate within this institution and I plan to stay so."

A few historians and historic players have put the history of psychosurgery and especially its excesses in context, notably Elliot S. Valenstein in *Great and Desperate Cures,* David Shutts in *Lobotomy,* and Samuel I. Shuman in *Psychosurgery and the Medical Control of Violence.* Their views are cited in the text and bibliography and I have relied heavily and gratefully on them and others for details and perspective. But most reviews of that era are relentlessly vague, unforgiving, or both—positions once justified, but now vulnerable to new knowledge and rising demands for help from the mentally ill and their advocates. Moreover, practically nothing has been written to update the general public in the last ten years about the new operations, their availability, and the ongoing problems they pose.

People must still ask who can and should benefit from surgery? How can such procedures best be regulated? Under what circumstances can an irreversible procedure be justified in patients who may never be able to give informed consent to their own treatment? Can doctors protect treatments aimed at relieving a person's suffering from being diverted to the control of behaviors and ideas that are unpleasant, aberrant, or undesirable? Do those who want to expand psychosurgery reinforce the absurd notion that the mind is a machine run by software no less subject to analysis and repair than a PC program hit by a hacker's virus?

There are many who, for understandable reasons, never want to reopen these inquiries, even if the desperately ill might benefit. In 1989, a San Francisco psychiatrist who lived through the antipsychiatry movement of the 1970s and treated lobotomized patients whose personalities were destroyed, told me:

> The average American, I fear, really believes that if you can fix a computer, why not a brain. It's a dangerous kind of thinking that has come back in style along with those who are strong on law and order and accept without question the medical model of mental illness. It's the notion that if people behave in a bizarre way that is unpleasant or uncomfortable or scary to us, the humane thing is to do whatever it takes to cure it, even if the treatment is inhumane.

Or, as psychosurgery's harshest critic, Peter Breggin, once put it, "When somebody's at the end of his rope, do you hang him on it?"

Whatever point of view readers may bring to this story, I hope they agree that psychosurgery is a subject worth an open-minded look, if for no other reason than the lack of alternatives for thousands, perhaps millions, of mentally ill. "In the future as in the past," says psychiatrist Louis Jolyn West of the University of California at Los Angeles, "demand, born of great need, will drive the profession's interest and commitment to psychosurgery."

Today, as in the past, the need to balance treatment with protection from treatment abuse is especially important for the ill who are homeless, poor, female, and imprisoned as well as for children and minorities. I am mindful that they were historically the guinea pigs of psychosurgery and could become so again.

On the other hand, they could become beneficiaries of a therapy that still has promises to keep.

Psychosurgery

CHAPTER ONE

POOR AUNT JOAN

Only if you experienced how bad it was, only if you visited the snake pits that existed not too long ago for me to remember, can you understand why desperate measures were nurtured by our psychiatric institutions and accepted as moral.

—MELVIN SABSHIN, M.D., PAST PRESIDENT, THE AMERICAN PSYCHIATRIC ASSOCIATION

People who have never seen these patients cannot begin to understand how bad it was. There were no treatments and patients were unbelievably destructive. The only way to deal with them was locked doors and armed squads of guards. It's so easy to be critical now.

—DONLIN LONG, M.D., CHAIRMAN, DEPARTMENT OF NEUROSURGERY, THE JOHNS HOPKINS UNIVERSITY SCHOOL OF MEDICINE

Last year, surgeons worldwide performed hundreds, perhaps thousands, of operations on the brain to treat the mind, operations that permanently destroyed brain tissue in efforts to restore mental health. Precise statistics are impossible to obtain for all but a few dozen cases, an astonishing phenomenon in this age of modern science, but one that is emblematic. They must work without fanfare, these surgeons insist, because to do otherwise would draw irrational criticism from too many who don't, or won't, understand the need for these operations and whose misguided (in their opinion) efforts to protect the mentally ill in fact would deny such patients treatment that could salvage their minds and lives.

There is a great deal of truth in what these medical scientists say. On the other hand, two years of inquiry into modern psychosurgery suggests another explanation for the silence that surrounds the reemergence of these procedures in the United States, Europe, and elsewhere. It is the arrogant unwillingness of physicians and psychiatrists to share their knowledge or to risk having their power to operate further curbed by courts, regulators, hospital review boards, or patient advocate groups. That power needs some curbing; there are without question those who would use their knowledge and skill to control people who are "inconvenient," who behave and think abnormally or outside the mainstream, who disturb our peace. Their numbers are small, but their goals justifiably scary.

The unhappy further truth is that both explanations hold merit. But, more to the point, patients suffer the consequences of both the silence and the arrogance. The public's lack of access to information about these operations is appalling, leaving desperate patients and their families to go begging for help that may exist, but never comes.

Too many doctors are unwilling to face critics, rational or otherwise; to explain and share what they know; and to take responsibility for their actions. Like the medical community's lagging response to the so-called animal rights movement, doctors' response to psychosurgery's critics is, generally, to hide out, shoo them away, dismiss them as "nuts," or claim lack of precious time and resources to spend on "tilting at windmills." The results of such head-in-the-sand behavior with respect to the animal rights lobby have been skyrocketing costs for research, abandonment of some vital research altogether, and a growing Luddite, antiscience population so fearful of science's power that some are ready to give rats equal rights with people and sacrifice human health and lives to preserve pit bulls. Instead of recognizing the need to

reform some aspects of animal research, and respond to their critics with compassion *and* facts, the scientific community until very
recently fought back only with disdain and neglect. With respect
to modern psychosurgery, this kind of response has meant patients
who are abandoned, doctors who play safe, and scientific pursuits
without champions.

Why we've come to this sad state of affairs is rooted in medical
traditions and mystique, the historically high status afforded
physicians and surgeons, and a good dose of ignorance. But it also
is rooted in a mass experiment and experience that began about
sixty years ago.

In his 1987 autobiography, *The Education of a Yankee,* New
England editor/author Judson Hale recalls the story of one of his
mother's two young sisters, Joan Sagendorph. After a post-Thanks-
giving "coming out" in 1935, the lovely Boston debutante was "the
unlucky recipient of a lobotomy a couple of years later."
Lobotomies, Hale explained, "were a briefly popular medical procedure of the '30s in which one or more nerves attached to lobes
of the brain, those having to do with emotions in Aunt Joan's case,
were surgically severed." The lobotomy was performed on Aunt
Joan, his family reported,

> because of her emotionally overwrought state of mind (she threw a
> flowerpot at my maternal grandmother) after being stood up at her
> church wedding by a man who was already married. The operation
> rendered her incapable of leading a normal life outside of an institu-
> tion.... Because she was unfortunate enough to have been deceived by
> a married man and to have heaved a flowerpot at her mother at the
> precise time this particular medical fad was being practiced in the
> medical capital of the world (Boston) where she lived, Aunt Joan
> became for the rest of her life, poor Aunt Joan.

A more glossy, glib, passionless description of lobotomy is hard
to imagine. The grim reality is that between 1936 and 1960, an
estimated 50,000 mutilating lobotomies were performed in the
United States alone. Some profoundly psychotic patients were

helped, but needless damage was done to the minds and brains of schizophrenics and innocent victims like Aunt Joan, who may, at worst, have been neurotic.

Some 2,400 years earlier, Hippocrates condoned "extreme cures" for "extreme disease," but even he might have wavered over prefrontal lobotomies and their surgical relatives. Consider the work of just one psychosurgeon, Walter Freeman, America's preeminent lobotomist and the operation's most ardent advocate.

It is January 1946, in an office on R Street in Washington, D.C. The flamboyant, goateed Freeman, a professor of neurology at George Washington University but not a certified surgeon, had become impatient and dissatisfied with prefrontal lobotomies in which the skull was cut open, or holes drilled in it so that massive amounts of brain tissue could be scooped out with a blunt, metal, spatulalike instrument or killed with alcohol injections. All that "opening" took too long, in Freeman's opinion, and required a hospital and surgical team. So now, after a few hours of tests on cadaver brains, he used an ice pick supplied by the Uline Ice Company, and did the first of thousands of transorbital lobotomies on a woman named Ellen.

Compare Hale's sanitized narrative with a letter Freeman wrote to his son describing the new operation: "I have been trying," he wrote, a procedure that

> consists of knocking [patients] out with an [electric] shock and while they are under the "anesthetic" thrusting an ice pick up between the eyeball and eyelid through the roof of the [bony] orbit [or eye socket around the eyeball] actually into the frontal lobe of the brain and making the lateral cut by swinging the thing from side to side. I have done now two patients on both sides and another on one side without running into any complications except a very black eye in one case. There may be trouble later on but it seemed fairly easy, although definitely a disagreeable thing to watch.

By 1948, Freeman apparently decided that if some mutilated frontal lobe was good, more of this "disagreeable thing" was better. Instead of moving the handle of the ice pick, or "leukotome" (from the Greek for "white matter" and "cutting instrument"), only side to side, he now forced the handle upward, driving the tip into deeper parts of the frontal lobe. In a 1958 play called *Suddenly, Last Summer,* Tennessee Williams dramatized for all time the terror lobotomy posed, but even Williams could not have improved on the chilling specter Freeman's own description of the operation evokes to this day:

> After two to five successive electroconvulsive shocks ... to maintain a state of coma for about five minutes [and] when the last convulsion subsides, the nurse places a towel over the nose and mouth to prevent contamination by saliva or nasal secretions. I pinch the upper eyelid ... and bring it away from the eyeball. I then insert the point of the trans-orbital leukotome into the conjunctival sac [around the white part of the eyeball] ... and move the point around until it settles against the vault of the orbit. I then drop to one knee beside the table in order to aim the instrument parallel with the bony ridges of the nose and tap the handle to drive it through the orbital plate [the back of the eye socket] to a depth of five centimeters. The handle is then pulled as far [to the side] as the rim of the orbit will permit. I then return the instrument half way to its previous position and drive it further to a depth of seven centimeters.... Again, I sight the instrument and take a profile photograph. This is the nearest approach to precision of which the method can boast.... Then comes the ticklish part. Arteries are within reach. Checking to make certain that the instrument is still parallel to the bony ridge of the nose, the handle is moved 20 degrees medially and 30 degrees laterally. The deep front cut followed: Standing behind the head of the patient I strongly elevate the handle of the instrument in this oblique plane until the shaft lies as nearly as possible parallel with the orbital plate and then the handle is returned to the mid position. The instrument is withdrawn, applying pressure on the upper eyelid to control escape of blood and ... fluid. I then proceed with the opposite side [with a sterile second instrument].... In some instances, when the ... leukotome is thrust through the orbital plate with a mere tap of the knuckle, there is no difficulty at all; in other cases, however, the plate is so thick and heavy that the operator risks bending or breaking the instrument. Quite often there is a sudden give or even an audible crack as the ... plate fractures.

Not surprisingly, the procedure sickened most who watched it, including veteran clinicians. According to historian Elliot S. Valenstein, one 74-year-old doctor fainted and Freeman was reportedly fond of saying he was "as good as Frank Sinatra" in getting young people to pass out.

Unmoved by squeamish stomachs, Freeman developed a huge private practice in Washington, D.C., and soon took his show on the road, operating on depressed, anxious, phobic, paranoid, "frigid," homosexual, hyperactive, delusional, violent, neurotic, psychotic, and schizophrenic patients. No brain, no mind, was sacrosanct. Most patients, he claimed, were up in a day or two, "relaxed," sick to their stomachs for a bit, disoriented for a little while, but suffering little more than a telltale black eye.

This is what psychosurgery *really* was, in its most extreme and widespread form. And although refinements, caution, and general anesthesia made some of the operations Freeman's colleagues performed in the 1930s, 1940s, and 1950s somewhat less ghastly and less destructive, his procedures make it easy to understand the disgust psychosurgery still provokes.

Today, Freeman's barbaric prefrontal and transorbital leukotomies are long buried beside beatings and chains in the battle against mental illness. But psychosurgery remains a metaphor for the abuse of psychiatry and patients, based as it was on profound ignorance of the brain exceeded only by the profound arrogance of its perpetrators. Psychosurgeons in those days killed patients, crippled patients, cruelly damaged brains and personalities, and operated casually on large numbers of "Aunt Joans," whose ailments were no more psychotic than a broken heart. In doing so, they ensured that no matter the benefit to some—even many—people would forever cringe at the thought of such therapy.

Given their gruesome nature and the dubious, overstated outcomes, why did such operations come on the scene at all, much less prevail for so long? They were not, after all, the province of hacks or backwater psychiatric hospitals. They seduced the era's best psychiatrists, surgeons, and institutions.

The fairest response is that lobotomy erupted as a treatment of choice because life for the chronically mentally ill of that time—

and for their families—was relentlessly appalling. In the decades before the first of the major tranquilizers and mood-altering drugs were discovered, there was nothing to calm the terror, the violence, the despair that marked mental illness. As awful as lobotomies now seem to us, they were at the time arguably the lesser of the two evils. Those who underwent psychosurgery represented but a fraction of the hopelessly mentally ill—psychotics, schizophrenics, brain-damaged patients, many war veterans—confined in modern Bedlams, locked away in prison asylums, and hidden away in relatives' back rooms and in back wards for decades.

Frustrated, overworked, undereducated caretakers slapped them, spit on them, shackled them, or straitjacketed them for weeks or months at a time. Schizophrenics, by several estimates, filled 75 percent of state hospital beds and mentally ill children and adults took one of every two general hospital beds.

According to medical historian David Shutts, "the number of first admissions to psychiatric hospitals had grown at an alarming average rate of 80 percent a year during the 1930s." By 1936, the year of the first reported lobotomy, he reported "there was a total of 432,000 psychiatric patients in state hospitals in the United States alone. Although hospitalization for mood disorders (depression, anxiety) showed the most dramatic surge, there was also a significant rise in the number ... admitted for dementia praecox or schizophrenia," marked by irrationality, delusions, and paranoia. "The prognosis ... for ... schizophrenics was nearly hopeless ... leading to permanently demented states. Thus, most ... spent years, even decades, in psychiatric institutions, receiving little if any therapy and existing in what was predominantly a custodial environment."

What treatments existed were few and often both literally and figuratively shocking: Electrical currents and high doses of insulin and Metrazol (pentylenetetrazol) jarred depressed and hallucinating patients' brains. Some were helped, but many suffered fractures of bones in their thighs, spines, arms, jaws, and even hips, along with pain, brain damage, chemical poisoning, and terror.

Depressed patients, all considered suicide risks, were subject to mechanical restraints, barred windows, and a jaillike existence, relieved only by wet packs, baths, sedatives, and bouts of talk therapy.

"Mental hospitals were snakepits," says psychiatrist Melvin Sabshin. "In my career, I've visited places in Bangladesh that weren't that bad—filthy, overcrowded places. After you've seen that, you understand how natural it was to try anything that held a glimmer of hope of getting people out of those institutions. The thinking was the same as if today someone in desperate straits from cancer or some other disease needed help and doctors used sickening and potentially lethal drugs, accepting mighty risks. It was a risk-benefit gestalt."

Overlaying all of this were the turf battles of the caretakers: Psychiatrists saw abnormal personality as their battleground; yet neurologists claimed the field for study of the brain and nerves. The two camps moved back and forth across the neuropsychiatric war zones with little to guide their diagnoses or treatments. As historian Shutts put it:

> It was not unlikely for a neurologist in the 1930s to have as many as 70 percent of his patients suffering from purely psychiatric disorders, while psychiatrists—particularly those working in state hospitals—confronted neurological disorders such as arteriosclerosis, syphilis and alcoholism in well over half of their patients.... Most psychiatrists were so resolute in [blaming] psychological forces to a patient's behavior that they played down the relevance of even obvious organic symptoms. The inverse of this medical arrogance was true of most neurologists, who asserted that a physical abnormality of the nervous system was the causative factor in a majority of cases of mental illness. Consequently, neurologists and psychiatrists regarded each others' treatments as an expensive waste of effort and often declined to send their patients to one another for consultation.

While a few doctors such as biological psychiatrist Adolph Meyer at Johns Hopkins were beginning to sort out the relative responsibilities of biology and psychology in the diagnosis and treatment of mental illness, patients and their families suffered.

Meyer himself introduced insulin shock therapy and lobotomy to the Hopkins faculty with cautious, but hopeful, praise. The time was ripe for something—anything—new that would cut across disciplines and bring relief to patients and the medical community alike.

Against this backdrop came the vision of Portuguese neurologist Antonio Egas Moniz. In 1936, he first reported that he had cut into the brain lobes of patients with uncontrollable emotional disease, especially but not only schizophrenia, in a heroic effort to cure them. The new formula for Sabshin's psychiatric gestalt was right there between the lines of his scholarly presentation at an international scientific meeting.

Moniz's idea was extreme, but not particularly original. Indeed, the history of psychosurgery can trace its roots to prehistoric attempts at trepanning by the Incas and other primitive tribes who believed that evil spirits could be evicted from the mind and soul, and mental illness cured, by creating openings in the brain to let them out. Early Romans had observed that insanity was occasionally cured by a sword wound to the head, what might now be called accidental psychosurgery.

The frontal lobes as a theoretical target for surgery in fact emerged after such "accidental" lobotomies, notably the case of a young dynamite worker, Phineas Gage, in 1848. Gage had survived a severe head injury sustained when the force of an explosion pushed an iron rod through his left cheek and up into the frontal lobes of his brain. Gage had, by all accounts, been an intelligent and easy-going man, but, after his wound healed, became impulsive, irritable, unreliable, and antisocial.

The modern roots of psychosurgery reach to the 1880s, when Gottlieb Burckhardt, a Swiss psychiatrist with his own mental hospital, removed pieces of cortex in order, he wrote, "to extract from the brain mechanism the emotional and impulsive element" and calm agitated patients. An Estonian surgeon, Lodivicus Puusepp, tried three similar operations in 1910, but abandoned the idea.

All of these attempts were essentially "blind" operations,

because there were no means of seeing inside the brain. But by 1920, Hopkins neurosurgeon Walter Dandy had developed X-ray techniques to outline the brain's main cavities, and in 1932, he unintentionally advanced the case for psychosurgery when he removed a life-threatening brain tumor from the frontal lobes of a 39-year-old stockbroker, Joe A. Describing Joe A., neurologist Richard Brickner noted his lack of restraint, boastfulness, anger and aggression, euphoria, lack of initiative, impaired short-term memory, and lack of common sense. Joe recovered many of his intellectual abilities after the surgery, but was completely unable to function in his old life with an IQ of about 80 or 90. Astonishingly, the reaction to Joe's case was not horror at his brain damage, but avid interest in the evidence it provided that the frontal lobes were indeed the "seat of personality."

In 1933, Carlyle Jacobsen and his mentor, John Fulton, the chairman of Yale University's Department of Physiology and a protégé of Harvey Cushing, added immensely to that evidence and provided the next bit of rationale for the conceptual leap to psychosurgery. In an effort to create "experimental neurosis" in animals, they trained, or conditioned, chimpanzees to be angry, violent, and frustrated by having their keepers change the rules and rewards for good performance.

Eventually, they decided to see what the effects would be of frontal lobotomy on two of the chimps, Becky and Lucy. Before surgery, the animals displayed the usual frustrations. After, they did not seem to care, but were calm and passive. Becky, to be more specific, no longer responded to her mistakes and lack of treats with temper tantrums, although Lucy continued to display some anger. (A similar use of animals became infamous years later when Yale University's Dr. José Delgado used remote electrical stimulators in the frontal lobes of an enraged bull to stop it in its tracks.) Fulton and Jacobsen concluded that frontal lobe loss produced erratic and unpredictable influences on learning and behavior. But the experiments on Becky and Lucy seriously impressed an aging Portuguese neurologist who had made important contributions to the field of brain imaging in the development of cerebral angiography using radioactive dyes.

In 1935, the urbane and politically active Antonio Caetano de Abrere Freire, known as Egas Moniz (a name he assumed to shield his family from retribution for his antimonarchical activities), attended the Second International Neurological Congress in London and heard reports of the chimp experiments.

Accounts of what happened next vary. Clearly, Moniz went beyond Fulton's and Jacobsen's conclusions and believed the experiments showed without doubt that complete removal of the frontal lobes calmed and pacified the animals, reducing their anxiety, neurosis, and anger. And he concluded that the experiments were applicable to people. Somewhere along the line, Moniz decided to systematically wound the brain, making him the putative "father" of psychosurgery.

In Fulton's version of the story, Moniz startled and upset him at the London meeting with the suggestion that the Becky and Lucy experiments—particularly Becky's surgically induced "happiness"—might help depressed humans. (Later, actually, Fulton rushed to tout psychosurgery, recruiting his vast network of top neurosurgeons and neuroscientists to its value, including Drs. Henry Viets, Percival Bailey, Harry Solomon, and Paul Bucy. Lending further credence to Moniz's claim to the "discovery" of psychosurgery, Science Service distributed a press release about his prolobotomy lectures at Mayo and other medical schools. He used personal connections to quash criticism in the popular press, including negative comments from the New York Academy of Medicine solicited by a writer for the *Saturday Evening Post*.)

In fact, Moniz may already have known about Becky and Lucy by the time he went to the London congress and may already have been thinking about a less drastic form of operation, a lobotomy (or leukotomy) for treating depressed or violent patients. Critics say Moniz stole the idea, while his champions claim he had already thought it up and The London Congress just affirmed his idea.

In any event, as one observer put it, "the shot fired" by Fulton into Becky's frontal lobes was indeed heard round the world, first, probably, by Moniz and his neurosurgeon, Almeida Lima, who performed the first lobotomy on a woman patient on November 12, 1936. The 63-year-old former prostitute had syphilis, mania, depression, and anxiety and displayed paranoid behavior. Two months after her operation, Moniz considered her cured and the following year, 1937, he reported on 20 psychotics and neurotics, all of whom had the same operation: a cut across the whole top of the cortex in the front of the brain. He claimed cure for one-third of his patients, improvement for one-third, and status quo for the remaining third.

Moniz, who was not a psychiatrist, credited the success of lobotomy to his theory that mental illness was caused by an abnormally "fixed" pattern of brain cell communications. Disrupting the pattern permanently would cure the illness.

Even if his theory had been true, quipped one critic, his treatment was like "weeding a garden with a hand grenade." But neither Moniz nor his reputation suffered from his lack of scientific rigor or common sense. He had given the world a relatively quick, simple operation to help the hopeless, to empower the helpless psychiatric community.

In what many consider poetic justice, Moniz was shot and crippled by one of his patients, but not before word of his achievements spread, especially to the United States; between 1936 and 1954, lobotomy became the buzzword and bylaw of psychiatric practice. The chief American disciples were our old friend neurologist Freeman and his close colleague, neurosurgeon James Watts, who premiered the U.S. lobotomy on September 14, 1936, and produced the first textbook on the subject in 1942, called *Psychosurgery in the Treatment of Mental Disorders and Intractable Pain*. Both worked at George Washington University in Washington, D.C.

Exploiting the emerging work of neuroanatomists who were mapping the cortex, the pair performed literally thousands of "trial-and-error" operations. Instead of moving from careful experimental work on animals or waiting for knowledge of brain imaging to clearly illuminate their way and reduce potential damage, they used their patients the way today's neurosurgeons might use lab animals and sustained far less outrage than today's animal rights activists lob at medical researchers. Wrote one chronicler of these times, science writer David Noonan, "Freeman and Watts's faith in psychosurgery was absolute. They made it the center of their careers and in the process they systematically abused their patients, the power they wielded as doctors and even the existing knowledge of the brain and its functions."

By 1949, when to the astonishment of many Moniz won the Nobel Prize for his concept (Freeman nominated him), doctors already had performed some variety of psychosurgery on at least 25,000 to 30,000 American and 10,000 British patients.

The true number of patients operated on will never be known, but by the early 1950s, surgeons and psychiatrists were operating all over the United States and abroad, to the usually uncritical acclaim of the mass media, families of patients, and administrators of every major psychiatric institution and public and private hospital. *Reader's Digest, Time, Newsweek, Life, the New York Times,* and other publications made a media star of Freeman, who by then was operating on hundreds of people a year, sometimes several a day, taking less than ten minutes per procedure in wild displays of virtuosity with the leukotome.

He plunged his ice picks into brains everywhere, in 55 hospitals in 23 states, Canada, the Caribbean, and South America. From Little Rock, Arkansas, to Berkeley, California, and Lincoln, Nebraska, he apparently found the West and Midwest particularly receptive, according to his biographers. Once, in Iowa at Cherokee State Hospital, a leukotome accidentally sank up to the hilt when Freeman let go to take a picture. No matter. It was barely reported. In another case, Freeman called on a patient at a Silver Spring, Maryland, motel to find him unruly. Relatives grabbed the hapless man, and held him on the floor while Freeman gave him electric shocks from a portable kit he carried. Then, wrote a colleague who heard the story from Freeman, "it ... occurred to him [Freeman] that since the patient was already unconscious and he had a set of leukotomes in his pocket, he might just as well do the transorbital lobotomy right then and there. The patient did well."

Another time at the Sykesville State Hospital in Maryland, he tried to operate on a woman with paranoia and hallucinations who attacked people violently. He failed after the instrument broke into three pieces. One piece cut the woman's retina, blinding her. Undaunted, even after a second failure, he used a tougher instrument and rendered her, in his words "calm and accessible."

Freeman's by now famous impatience finally led him to an ambidextrous, two-fisted procedure, in which he shoved a leukotome through each eye socket before stepping behind for his "deep cut." As Valenstein described it, "He would grasp the two handles, one in each hand, and simultaneously force them upward.... After a long surgical session, his hands were often tender from the pressure."

The press ate it up.

As comforting as it would be to say so, however, the truth is that psychosurgery was not some mad scientist's cruel experiment, but a response to desperation. Psychosurgery arose and gained incredible popularity because of the abysmal record of treating, controlling, and relieving the suffering of mental patients; because of the intense interest of some of the world's greatest neurologists, psychiatrists, and neurosurgeons; and because of a social order in the 1920s and 1930s marked by national upheavals, war, and the twin stresses of industrialization and urbanization. The world, it seemed, was going mad and science was at the same time inventing the tools to test the fervently held beliefs that mental illness, violence, misery, and antisocial behavior were rooted in the brain cells and curable.

With legions of melancholy, agitated, fearful, violent, and bizarre patients, imagine the impact of a group of procedures that respected practitioners said would cure 30, 40, or 50 percent of patients, empty hospitals, and do it fast.

There were no objective diagnoses, no positron emission tomography (PET) scanners, no support groups, no patient advocacy or patient rights groups. The highly sensitized legal, social, and ethical environments that surround medical practice today were not yet in place and accountability in the medical establishment would not really come until government financing and regulation grew strong in the 1970s.

Whatever anger and horror we may feel now over the "poor Aunt Joans," those feelings were then overshadowed by the plight of patients without hope. Donlin Long, chief of neurosurgery at Hopkins Hospital, spends his workdays probing gently and deftly among brain cells with the aid of modern technology and clear maps of the brain. But he remembers a different time, at the University of Minnesota School of Medicine, where he did his surgical residency at the tail end of psychosurgery's "Golden Age."

"I remember one patient in particular," he said.

> She was a young, very attractive woman with small kids who was unbelievably phobic about dirt of any kind. She could not leave her bedroom or bathroom because everything she touched had to be washed. So if she wanted to open the door to her bedroom, first she had to open the door to the bathroom and wash her hands and the doorknob on the bedroom door, and in order to do that she had to touch the faucet and turn it on. So then she had to wash that before she could move on. She couldn't get anywhere at all. No one had been able to help her.

Kenneth Livingston, then the chief of neurosurgery at Minnesota, performed, "with the woman's fervent consent," Long notes, a lobotomy. "He turned her from a totally disabled person into a fully functioning wife and mother," Long says. "No, she was not someone you'd want to manage the family fortune. Some intellectual and reasoning function were lost, but she was joyful at her new life. All other treatments had failed completely. We were grateful for psychosurgery."

Livingston's patient was one among a large group of psychiatrically crippled people with obsessive-compulsive disorder (OCD), a condition well known in psychosurgery's early days, but not at all understood. Today (see Chapter 6) the genetic and biochemical roots of OCD are the subjects of intense and fruitful study. Drugs that target and sabotage biochemical receptors in the brain help many OCD patients. Delicate brain surgery helps others. But 50 years ago, suicide was too often the only way out of it.

Victims spent days and nights doing the same "ritual" acts over and over. One person might wash her hands for more than 10 hours a day, seven days a week, for 30 years. Another patient, treated by psychiatrist Michael Jenike of Harvard, showered for 8 hours a night. Another brushed his teeth for an hour or more each day, having to get up hours early to prepare for a normal workday and ever fearful of succumbing to multiple obsessions that would destroy his career. (The worst case Jenike said he ever saw was a woman in her 40s who had spent up to 13 hours a day washing her hands and house. She described her life as "hell," and no wonder. "Before she could use the soap she had to use some bleach on the soap to make sure the soap was clean. Before that, she had to use Ajax on the bleach bottle. If she happened to bump the edge of the sink while doing this, this would set off another hour and a half, two hours of ritual. She didn't really think there were germs there. It was just a feeling.")

For mental health workers, the job was a workday sentence in their patients' hell. Destruction and arson, for example, were everyday facts of life. The case literature is full of such accounts as that of the patient in a Minnesota state mental hospital who set fires in the pocket of her mother's apron, in her guardian's dressing gowns, and in the hospital where she had been confined for decades. Seven people died in the fires she set. (A bilateral amygdalotomy reportedly reduced her aggressive behavior without any loss of short-term memory or other debilitating side effects of lobotomy and finally ended her career as a firebug.)

In addition to OCD patients were many who functioned part of the time outside of institutions, but who became the "revolving door" populations of the state mental hospitals of the 1940s and 1950s and the homeless psychotics decades later. Often, they were the victims of the bipolar or manic-depressive psychosis.

These days, lithium and other drugs control the often violent mood swings that send the afflicted from super-energy highs to suicidal depths. Many patients function at a superior level during their "highs" and such victims as director Josh Logan and author Kate Millett have publicly celebrated both their conditions and their treatments. But before lithium, they and a less-famous population of manic depressives went in and out of hospitals several times a year, while their desperate families and doctors spent decades trying to keep the lid on.

Perhaps the most desperate—and numerous—cases of all the mentally ill who drove the engine of psychosurgery were schizophrenics. There are an estimated 45 million schizophrenics worldwide today, but experts believe the rate has been constant at about 1 percent of the population over the last century. Ironically, schizophrenia responded least of all the psychoses to psychosurgery, but its terrible and progressively worsening symptoms fueled the determination of psychosurgeons to help its victims.

"Franz" is a textbook case of that era. At 23, he told people he was a "riddle of bones." He heard buzzing noises, penetrating squeals, and voices with messages he sometimes understood but could not remember. He saw flashes of light and shadow in the middle of the room. Strangers, he said, sent their shadows to visit him in bed. He tasted soap in his mouth and absorbed poison from the bedpost. He chewed his tie, hoarded garbage, sat in a stupor for weeks, and hit his nurses. Occasionally he clowned and walked on his hands.

Schizophrenia's symptoms vary over time, but most patients wind up with some combination of hallucinations, delusions, paranoia, and disembodied voices talking to them.

First described in great detail in 1906 by a Swiss physician named Eugen Blueler, schizophrenia is characterized by broken or disordered thinking. The word *schizophrenia,* coined by Blueler from the Greek for "split mind," recognizes that the minds of schizophrenics operate not as integrated systems, but in bits and pieces that distort reality, muddy perceptions, and loosen the links between thoughts. Over time, victims confuse fantasy with reality for longer and longer periods. They make peculiar movements, giggle at tragedy, go for decades without speaking, and deteriorate in every single case, even with today's medications.

The famed dancer Nijinksy, one of Blueler's patients, had typical grandiose delusions, once writing, "I am God, Nijinsky is God.... All that I write is necessary to mankind." Diagnosed in 1919 at the age of 29, he never danced again. Patients like Nijinksy have given support to the popular notion that schizophrenics are often creative. Novelist Mark Vonnegut's autobiographical *Eden Express* tried to make that case. But those who are familiar with and treat the disease know better. "Anyone who has worked with schizophrenics for even a few weeks knows that there is nothing joyous, positive, romantic, or productively creative about this disease," according to Solomon Snyder, award-winning professor of psychiatry and neuroscience at Hopkins and an authority on the brain chemistry of schizophrenia and other diseases. "It destroys lives."

In the days before drugs controlled symptoms for at least some patients for a while, large populations of schizophrenics were confined to asylums and hospitals, tortured and disturbed by massive delusions and hallucinations, often requiring restraints and locked rooms to keep them and their behavior contained. Unable often to toilet themselves, stay groomed, eat a meal, or relate to anyone, these men and women became, literally, crazier and crazier. Many could not communicate their pain, for just as schizophrenia breaks up the mind's unity, so it distorts speech patterns, resulting in what psychiatrists call clang associations, word salads, or neologisms, a mental jumble of odd speech patterns that absolutely guarantee isolation from all normal human communication. One patient's word salad makes the point:

Well, when he was first bit on the slit on the rit and the man on the ran or the pan on the band and the sand on the man and the pan on the ban on the can on the man on the fan on the pan ... that's to keep the boogers from eating the woogers. Well it was a jigger and a figger and a figger and a bigger and men, and I'll swap you for a got you and a fair-haired far for a bar and jar for tar and rang dang ting tang with a be shag, he shag.

Sometimes, doctors, nurses, and relatives heard this kind of "talk" all day long.

Leonard Henson, director of adult psychiatry at the University of Minnesota medical center, remembers one 26-year-old male schizophrenic who, after 6 years of delusions, struck himself and put out his own eye. Kept in four-point restraints, he was given electroconvulsive therapy (ECT) once a week to keep him a little under control. No drugs helped him. "He was like most patients we saw in the 1940s and 1950s," Henson said. Eventually, he had a cingulotomy and amygdalotomy and is now calm and in a regular mental hospital. He still has schizophrenia, but he reads, learns, and is Henson says, "an enjoyable guy." That's the kind of patient for whom psychosurgery was viewed as a miracle.

Coping with madness is taxing, even for psychiatrists, and some doctors and families avoid or abandon schizophrenic patients. That's why in Aunt Joan's time, tens of thousands of patients were warehoused. They shuffled about, unsmiling, keening, wailing, throwing themselves and objects around, speaking gibberish, pacing constantly, flicking lit cigarettes, and complaining incessantly.

Violent and aggressive patients were even less well tolerated. Neurosurgeons Vernon Mark and William Sweet and psychiatrist Frank Ervin, in a 1972 book, *Violence and the Brain,* made an articulate case for using psychosurgery on certain kinds of violent behavior, a case that made them pariahs among civil rights leaders and social reformers and drove them from careers and even their home base in Boston. But the book documents the kind of patients for whom little else could be done without rendering them comatose with drugs or confining them to locked rooms.

One was Clara T. At 62, she had been a victim for 29 years of temporal lobe epilepsy after a head injury sustained in a fall on a patch of ice. Her seizures were accompanied by nausea and a sense of impending doom. Despite medications, her seizures were frequent. Her memory had failed and she physically assaulted anyone who came near her, biting and scratching delivery boys and her husband. On one occasion, when she was hospitalized, subduing a violent assault took four nurses and two male orderlies 45 minutes.

Another was Thomas R. a 34-year-old engineer, who flew unpredictably into uncontrollable rages, mostly at his wife. Convinced she was having an affair with a neighbor, her denials triggered frenzy. Clara and Thomas had psychosurgery, and in 1979 as we'll see in Chapter 7 Thomas was the trigger for a celebrated malpractice suit against the surgeons as well as the central character in Michael Crichton's best-seller, *The Terminal Man*.

In addition to schizophrenics, patients with OCD, the depressed and manic, the chronically panicked, and the explosively violent were patients in immense emotional distress as a result of unbearable physical pain and from depression so awful that the afflicted repeatedly attempted suicide. In the years before Prozac, tricyclic antidepressants, and other drugs, the melancholia was so deep these people remained in virtual trances, consumed by black thoughts for months, years, even decades. They grew obese, slept around the clock, fell into unpredictable fits of tears and ceaseless sobbing. Those who stayed out of hospitals numbed their pain with alcohol or other drugs. Some of the most dramatic descriptions of psychosurgeries in the 1940s and 1950s were accompanied in textbooks by "before" and "after" photos of intractably depressed patients. Before surgery, their faces were set in grief, eyes glazed, devoid of animation or the least hint of contentment. After, they are pictured with smiles that reach their eyes.

Not all psychosurgery was inspired by obviously "crazy," dangerous, or desperate cases. Some was aimed at socially or morally unacceptable behavior, especially sexual behavior, veiled in the cloak of "mental illness." It was in this domain that women, adolescents, children, the poor, and minorities were particularly victimized.

Victorian psychiatry had concocted elaborate theories of links between female psychosis and reproductive and sexual functions. Practitioners and theorists were convinced that women were particularly susceptible to mental disease because of pregnancy, childbirth, lactation, menstruation, and menopause. Men did not escape either: Rapists, pedophiles, homosexuals, exhibitionists, and transvestites were all candidates for lobotomies.

While the Victorians and their immediate successors were light-years off base, the practical and genuine problems faced by asylum superintendents and families caring for psychotic women and men were indeed exacerbated by sexual needs and behavior. Written descriptions by observers were vivid. Patients could be promiscuous, with multiple pregnancies and terrifying labor and delivery experiences. Rapes occurred and masturbation was so frequent and insistent that daily needs went unattended. Personal hygiene suffered, almost to extinction in some patients, and behavior that challenged every social norm kept the patients locked away.

Nothing, it seemed, could stop the lobotomy juggernaut, or its apologists. Enthusiasm far outstripped suspiciously bloated results. In a 1949 *Newsweek* article, the director of the New York State Psychiatric Institute of Columbia Presbyterian Medical Center complained of the "number of zombies that these operations turn out," but if anyone was listening, it was of little interest to lobotomists. In a later, 1950 edition of their text, Freeman and Watts claimed total victory for prefrontal lobotomy. Reporting on a total of 617 operations done mostly for schizophrenia (329), psychotic depression (147), and obsessive neurosis (121) (about 20 were done for pain), they pronounced 45 percent overall had good outcomes, 33 percent fair, and 19 percent poor, with 40 deaths after the immediate postoperative period. Exactly what "good," "fair," and "poor" stood for remains unclear to this day. Giants in the field of neuropsychiatry embraced psychosurgery almost in spite of themselves. Meyer, for example, a pioneer in biological psychiatry who was revolutionizing care of the mentally ill at the Johns Hopkins Hospital, said in one account of Freeman's earliest work, "I am not antagonistic to this work but find it very interesting. I have some of those hesitations about it that are mentioned by other discussants but ... the available facts are sufficient to justify the procedure in the hands of responsible persons."

The "verdict" of Freeman's colleagues was like opium to an addict and he went merrily on to further develop the faster, easier (for the surgeon) ice-pick procedures. Even his partner, Watts, a well-established neurosurgeon, was horrified at the careless risks posed by the new operation.

Bad reports had filtered in almost from the start of psychosurgery's rapid rise—reports of bleeding, suicide, further deterioration of IQ, inertia, sexual aberrations, pathological hunger, and aggressive behavior. Freeman himself admitted that the personality was flattened and altered and that their more radical operations on young people "were followed by prolonged inertia and incontinence" and by unsatisfactory results and platoons of "wax dummies" who lay immobile for weeks or months postoperatively.

A. Earl Walker, a former chief of neurosurgery at the University of Maryland School of Medicine now retired in New Mexico, tried in 1944 to evaluate the results of lobotomies in different hospitals and asylums, to find common ground in the case reports and thereby make some judgments. He found success rates all confoundingly varied and concluded that what probably accounted for the success or failure of any patient was the severity of illness of the patient to begin with, not any differences in the surgeries themselves, how they were done, who did them, or even *whether* they were done.

What was or was not the "improvement" attributed to psychosurgery was anybody's guess without rigorous standards of diagnosis and evaluation, both of which were nonexistent and most unwelcomed by Freeman and his disciples.

The reported "improvement" rates were also biased by the fact that there were no standard diagnostic criteria for selecting psychosurgery patients. Some surgeons did them on very sick patients, whatever that meant, while Freeman and Watts often did them "prophylactically." And who knows how many patients listed as "discharged home" went home because their families could handle them more humanely than the hospital after lobotomy. Freeman never once described any control group against which he compared diagnosis or treatment and those few carefully controlled studies that were done in the 1960s found no better outcome when lobotomy was compared with other treatments.

The almost total absence of scientific methodology in the evaluation of patients was noted bitterly in a 1946 speech to the American Psychiatric Association by psychologist Ward Halstead: "Not a single patient," he said, "had been adequately studied. For the moral and social responsibility to do this, there has been substituted a phenomenal array of case statistics. Unfortunately, the pyramiding of unknowns is scarcely a pathway to knowledge."

Data supporting the abuses and failures of psychosurgery continued to mount into the 1950s and 1960s:

- At Stanford University, a 1965 evaluation of 40 hospitalized male chronic schizophrenics—22 of whom had a bilateral prefrontal lobotomy 9 to 14 years earlier—found that fewer of those operated on could finish a multiple choice test and those who had the operation made more repeated errors of all kinds than those who had had no operation.

- A 1968 report in the *Journal of Nervous and Mental Disorders* found that all 74 psychotic patients operated on between 1940 and 1950 remained hospitalized and that convulsive seizures of the major motor type developed postoperatively in half of them.

- A study reported by the Ontario Department of Public Health in Toronto and the Canadian Medical Association on

116 patients—mostly demented, delusional schizophrenics—who had prefrontal lobotomies between 1948 and
1952 found that in 92 percent there were "late, serious personality defects, limited capacity for new learning and lack
of ability to plan or deal flexibly with a changing situation."

• A ten-year follow up of 134 men after lobotomy found
"nearly half disabled by seizures and a fourth by severe
intellectual impairment; fewer than 10 percent could leave
the hospital."

Despite the fact that some of the nation's best surgeons, psychiatrists, and institutions were up to their leukotomes in lobotomy
patients, the scientific output was wretched. One case in point
comes from two of the nation's preeminent neurosurgeons of that
time, James L. Poppen and Harry Solomon, and work that was
done at the famed Lahey Clinic in Boston and the Boston Psychopathic Hospital.

Historian Valenstein has written that Solomon waxed poetic
about the improvements he saw in lobotomized patients compared with earlier patients, but "presented no convincing evidence that patients during previous decades were comparable
with those selected for lobotomy. While the evidence, without
comparable non-surgical control subjects, had little scientific
value, the staff was apparently convinced and by 1950, more than
500 ... open lobotomies had been performed at the Boston Psychopathic Hospital [alone]." According to Valenstein, Solomon
claimed 40 percent of the chronically ill patients were sent home,
with 20 percent of that group pronounced relatively able to cope
with life. As for the remaining 60 percent, Solomon insisted they
lived a "more satisfying and contented life in institutions." There
was never an independent evaluation or standards of evaluation
applied to check those claims.

Even if scientists were to accept the overblown claims of
improvement provided by the foxes governing their own henhous-

es, the statistics had, in Valenstein's words, "no meaning without a truly comparable, unoperated comparison group. The implicit assumption behind the statistical data was that all or most of the patients would have progressively deteriorated, requiring institutionalization for the remainder of their lives if lobotomy had not been performed." That was the rationale behind operating on patients not only as a last resort, but also on those who were far less ill.

Just as damning was evidence that many patients *did* get better even in the "snakepit" days. Before the advent of psychosurgery or shock therapy, which was introduced in the 1930s, studies suggest that more than 40 percent of manic depressives eventually left the hospital and functioned well and another 27 percent were improved and discharged. A preeminent textbook on nervous disorders at the time, written by Drs. Smith Ely Jelliffe and William A. White in 1935, taught that long before *any* somatic treatments were available, simple rest, sedation, and support helped seven out of ten patents with severe depression, manic depressive psychosis, and disorders other than schizophrenia go home from the hospital better than they came in.

The outrageous abuses of psychosurgery highlighted in these stories did occur. But in their written records, Freeman and Watts also described in detail scores of patients they brought to their operating rooms and helped. Their accounts are, to be sure, biased by their heavy investment in the procedures. But even the sternest critics acknowledge that for many patients, psychosurgery was a godsend.

Patients like the 20-year-old who believed Jesus Christ, under the influence of unscrupulous men, was preventing him from following his own judgment; or the 59-year-old matron, sick for 35 years, who burned two overcoats because they were "contaminated" by a friend's touch. Doctors successfully treated a 19-year-old boy who hallucinated, kept his hands over his head, grimaced all the time, wrote letters to God, punched the air with his fists, and was uncontrollable at home; and the 36-year-old draftsman who believed he was followed constantly by the FBI, tried to commit suicide, and spent hours thinking about the devil.

"Lobotomy was a beginning," said Clyde Stanfield, a psychiatrist now at the Denver, Colorado, VA hospital medical center and a founding member of the Mt. Airy Psychiatric Center, where dozens of lobotomies were performed in the 1950s. In a lengthy interview, Stanfield pointed out that "lobotomy released some patients from prison or hospitals where they had been warehoused for decades. It meant taking responsibility, gambling on doing more harm than good.... But we had to do something if we could. Those were very desperate times."

Eventually, the lack of rigorous diagnosis, evaluation, and follow-up; the brutality of the ice-pick surgeries; the growing civil rights, bioethics, consumer, and patients rights movements; and the advent of the major neuroleptic drugs turned the promise of psychosurgery into an agony for the medical profession and psychiatric institutions.

By the 1970s, reporters were less awestruck and less inclined to accept the "miracle" cures and the risks. A science writer, Joel Greenberg, in a typical article for the *New York Times Magazine,* while describing modern psychosurgery in a Boston hospital, described board-certified surgeons, modern X-ray equipment, and tissue-sparing devices but reported no claims of instant cure. He quoted extensively from critics and reviewed the abuses of the past.

The freewheeling days of Freeman and Watts are gone and except in the rhetoric of those stridently against any physical treatment of mental illness, psychosurgery is no longer an uncontrolled threat. Yet the lessons are still painful for psychiatrists and neurosurgeons who lost professional autonomy, and the fear of abuse in the future is not altogether inappropriate. In our haste to treat, in our reliance on "modern" means that are less visibly brutal than ice picks, treatments of the mentally ill can still do damage. Drugs that control schizophrenics cause irreversible palsy. Valium and other antianxiety drugs are addictive. Prozac, the "wonder drug" of psychiatry in the 1980s, prescribed an estimated million times a month for patients suffering from depression, produces stunning results, but a report from Harvard Medical School in 1990 suggests that 7 to 8 percent of all those on Prozac may become violent or suicidal, injuring themselves or others.

If the first psychosurgeons had stuck to the worst cases, kept good records, proceeded carefully, reported honestly, learned as they went, and been more sensitive to their failures, psychiatry might not have lost its way in a quagmire of unethical and destructive operations and psychiatric patients like Aunt Joan much earlier would have won protections they needed.

Much has happened since Moniz's day that renders the "Aunt Joan" scenario moot. But these same events have hidden some compelling facts about psychosurgery as well, and driven interest in the procedures almost underground. The fact remains that the operations helped some people. Pychosurgery had then, and has now, the potential to help patients.

The time has come, perhaps, to face the past and the present, to uncover the interest and activity in neurosurgery for psychiatric disorder, to let the public in on what a small but growing number of doctors and patients know, and to encourage the advancement of knowledge while also protecting the helpless from abuse.

A first step is learning about those parts of the brain that define the mind and the consequences of damaging them.

CHAPTER TWO

TARGET OF THE KNIFE: THE PSYCHOLOGICAL BRAIN

From the brain, and from the brain only, arise our pleasures, joys, laughter and jests, as well as our sorrows, pains, griefs and tears. . . . It is the same thing which makes us mad or delirious, inspires us with dread or fears.

—HIPPOCRATES, FOURTH CENTURY B.C.

For those who drilled holes and plunged instruments into tens of thousands of brains, the target was feelings, not tissue; mind, not brain. Prefrontal lobotomies, and ultimately all psychosurgery, is designed to sever or untangle miswired connections, to alter the emotional and psychological operations of the organ of thought, not only—or necessarily—its biological disorders. History judged harshly the mutilations surgeons caused en route to their targets. But their persistence was driven by the conviction that there are separate anatomical sites in the brain tied to personality and behavior, distinct from thought and intellect.

As we've seen, neurologist Walter Freeman and neurosurgeon James Watts staked that claim in 1942 with hyperbolic glee. "With psychosurgery," they crowed in jacket copy for a textbook, "certain intellectual processes are revealed as running along without emotion ... when the connection between the frontal lobe and the thalamus is severed." Their work, they concluded, revealed no less than "how personality can be cut to measure, sounding a note of hope for those who are afflicted with insanity."

By 1950, Egas Moniz's Nobel Prize had become dramatic affirmation of the stakeholders' embrace of surgically tailored personalities. And what generated that embrace were precisely those connections Hippocrates conceived by intuition. Moniz, his surgeon Almeida Lima, and Freeman, their most ardent disciple, were after disordered minds, not diseased cells.

What Hippocrates divined and modern science later confirmed is the existence of their targets, the intricate network of delicate communications systems—some hard wired—in the limbic system or "emotional brain."

This is the part of the brain that governs feeling and some thought, motivation, and behavior. What doctors meant then—and mean now—when they say *psychosurgery* or *behavioral surgery* is removal, destruction, or disconnection of brain tissues with the specific intent of changing mood or behavior, with or without evidence of organic brain disease. The limbic system is not the thinking brain of problem solving, reading, writing, and arithmetic, but the primitive brain of instinct, fight or flight reactions, fear, eating, drinking, sexual behavior, autonomic regulation, and gland function.

Knowledge of the limbic system reveals and explains much about the past and present interest in psychosurgery, the determination of its advocates, the fear it evokes of mind control, and the ongoing controversy that surrounds even safe, modern versions. The reason is that within the limbic system are the tangible roots of what makes us essentially human.

Anyone who has experienced the everyday links between aging and memory, pain and pleasure, stress and physical illness, love and a rapid heart beat, pain and fear understands the lure of psychosurgery and the implications—good and evil—of this kind of therapy. If the "mindful" part of the brain actually connects with nerves, chemicals, and physical characteristics, then modifying one modifies one or more of the others as well. As Cornell University psychologist and author Michael S. Gazzaniga notes, the mind is not some free-floating thing separate from the brain, a set of "operating rules" that "push information around in such a fashion that the actual functioning of the nerves can be influenced by what the mind does." "What's remarkable about the anatomy of the brain," adds Haring Nauta of Johns Hopkins, "is that the anatomical systems that govern and operate our senses, movements and emotions are organized along very similar, parallel lines."

This means that limbic system circuitry has a lot in common with sensory and motor organization. "We are beginning to understand," Nauta says, "that if something is operating in one part of the [brain], the same *process* may take place in another, even if the outcomes vary. The boundaries are blurring between neurosurgery for treatment of such disorders as pain and Parkinson's disease and treatment of so-called purely psychological disorders. There are harmonies between parts of the brain and the systems that govern it."

Given the origin of the limbic system, none of this is surprising, because the limbic system is where mind and body first came together in evolutionary development; where nature forged the links between anxiety and rapid heart beats, sexual arousal, and sweat; where all the senses join and where emotional feelings are monitored and channeled to influence the body through its nervous system and glands.*

Scientists in an earlier time compared the limbic system to Sig-

---

*There are differences between these associations and psychosomatic illness, which reflects a different kind of link between emotions and disease. In psychosomatic illness, psychological factors are involved in the initiation or cause of damage to an organ or the way an organ works. Asthma, peptic ulcer, migraine headache, and high blood pressure often have psychosomatic origins. This does not mean, as many mistakenly believe, that the illness is "all in the head." In true psychosomatic illness, there is actual organic or functional damage. Thus patients who are hypochondriacs—obsessed with their bodily activities—often get physical symptoms, but have no physical manifestations of disease.

mund Freud's unconscious mind, the part of the brain that links feeling, thinking, and the senses; that is responsible for our emotional biases and what we call experience; that takes in a random, chaotic world and imposes order by applying what we've learned, what we feel, what we get pleasure or pain from, what we want and expect, and finally, guiding everything we eventually perceive and do. As mentioned earlier, the limbic system itself cannot think, but it is, ironically, responsible for what society deems to be rational and mentally normal. Thus it contains the couriers of our emotions, and disorders of the limbic system are at the foundation of what we call mental illness.

As British psychiatrist Desmond Kelly, who directs a psychosurgical clinic, points out, evolution eventually put the neocortex, or "new" higher brain functions in charge of more primitive, older structures concerned with intuition, fight, flight, smell, and emotional reactions to fear and pain. We're all more attentive these days to the parts of our brains that can do advanced algebra and read Plato. But everything that goes on in the limbic system to regulate mood, drive, and emotional reactions actually creates our conscious world, the "real" world we must deal with every day. The limbic system helps people sift, sort, and remember what brings them rewards and punishments. What goes wrong in the limbic system, with our minds, vastly influences what we do, how we think, and whether we function successfully.

Navigating and mapping all the neurological crossroads involved in psychiatric and behavioral abnormalities are a long way off. But in the limbic system, psychosurgeons of the past were confident they had found the right county. Today's neuroscientists are more sure of it.

Geographically, the limbic system is a group of brain structures and nerve circuits, buried deep in the temporal lobes on both sides of the brain, and forming a ring around the brain stem, or primitive brain. The front-most and upper limit of the limbic system is the cingulum, also referred to as the cingulate cortex, which nests against the prefrontal lobe and became the main targets of the prefrontal lobotomy. The frontal lobes modify and modulate the primitive limbic system. The classic prefrontal lobotomy of Freeman and Watts involved the indiscriminate division of as many fronto-limbic connections as possible, which often resulted in intellectual impairment, lack of self-control, euphoria, and agressive outbursts, as well as a 6 percent death rate.

The cingulate gyrus is on one of the major limbic circuits (called Papez) that link the septum to the hippocampus, mammillary body, thalamus, and back to the cingulate gyrus to close the loop. The cingulate gyrus is also on one of the major pathways by which the frontal lobe regulates limbic system function. The second limbic circuit is the so-called defense reaction circuit, that passes from the hypothalamus to amygdala and back to the hypothalamus. Electrical stimulation studies of these structures and their interconnections have shown behavioral changes associated with fight or flight. In some animal studies, the heart rate goes up, blood pressure rises, blood is diverted to muscle, and the animal adopts an aggressive posture, ready to fight or run away as if mortally threatened.

In short, these circuits, based around and in the cingulum, amygdala, mammillary body, thalamus, hypothalamus, and hippocampus, form the major functional or operations structures of the limbic system. They were the relay centers of nerve fibers that were the main target of destruction by Freeman and Watts.

The hippocampus is a bundle of fibers linked to learning and short-term memory. Along with the fornix, a stalk of nerves leading out of the hippocampus, it carries signals in and around the limbic system and forms electrochemical junctions for the emotional brain. Close by is the hippocampal gyrus, a big convolution, or groove, in the hippocampus that works with the frontal lobes, parts of the thalamus, and the hypothalamus to regulate emotional response. The hippocampus is also important in regulating the ability to concentrate or pay attention.

The amygdala, located in the lower arc of the limbic brain, is the seat of "fight or flight" reactions, and removal (amygdalectomy) or surgical lesions on this circuit (amygdalotomy) lead to profound behavior changes, especially with respect to violent behavior. The famous experimental psychologist José Delgado, for example, made aggressive, dominant bulls passive by damaging or damping down the animals' amygdala. There is some evidence that the amygdala also appears to have a major role in processing and recalling pleasant or painful consequences of experiences and damage to the amygdala may flatten or remove some major effects of this property.

Experimental electrical stimulation of various parts of the limbic system have both identified and guided surgery for areas of the brain involved in rage, anxiety, hyperactivity, hallucinations, obsessive-compulsive disorder, pain, violence, abnormal sexual behavior, spastic tremors, and a host of other psychological and behavioral conditions.

Some of the limbic system's structures have intricate nerve and chemical links within themselves and with higher (cortex) and lower (brain stem) areas of the brain. In this way, they form a crossroad for some of the intellectual and motor behavior activities of the brain that are connected with feelings, emotions, and stress, from rage and love to fear and panic.

The connections with the upper, more "intellectual" part of the brain primarily influence the way the brain sees, feels, and reacts to reality. For instance, they are responsible for the fact that when we smell the perfume worn by an unfaithful lover, the memory we recall and the feeling we feel is sad, not "neutral." Such connections are why anxiety can distort a mild threat (someone's grimace) into panic, or mild pain into anguish.

The limbic system's activities also help determine which part of our world we pay attention to and with how much intensity. How a dripping faucet may irritate us to distraction if we're upset, but become little more than unconscious background noise when we're not. Why editors in a noisy newsroom can blot out the usual chat, but will react immediately if an out-of-context sound—a child's cry—erupts.

Significantly, much of the limbic system also is heavy with chemical receptors, eager and waiting to be dosed with the chemicals of feeling and mood.

In recent years, neuroscientists have identified and analyzed more than 40 of these "neurotransmitters" that fit, like molecular keys in locks, into receptors on the surfaces of cells distributed around the brain. Among the best known neurotransmitters are acetylcholine, dopamine, endorphins, γ-aminobutyric acid (GABA), norepinephrine, and serotonin. When acetylcholine fails, Alzheimer's disease is one consequence, with its characteristic memory loss and sometimes hostile behavior. A lack of dopamine leads to Parkinson's disease, marked by tremors and muscle failure. When there is too much dopamine or too many receptors sucking up dopamine, schizophrenia may emerge.

Endorphins, the brain's own opiates, reduce or prevent perception of both physical and emotional pain. (The so-called runner's high is produced, apparently, by endorphin release.) GABA influences other neurotransmitters and is associated with aggressive behavior. Low levels of norepinephrine are closely linked to severe depression and possibly manic-depressive illness. Moreover, during panic and anxiety, the brain triggers the release of epinephrine (also called adrenaline), which results in an increase of heart rate and blood pressure and the diversion of blood from the skin to muscle to prepare the body automatically for that "fight or flight" response discussed earlier. An imbalance of serotonin is thought to be associated with severe depression, aggression, anorexia nervosa and other eating disorders, migraine, and insomnia.

Modern psychoactive drugs—such as tranquilizers, mood elevators, and antidepressants—suppress, enhance, or modify the activities of these brain chemicals to excite (cocaine, barbiturates, amphetamines), depress (alcohol, tranquilizers) and regulate (lithium, mood elevators, pain relievers) mood, thought, and emotions. Successful efforts, moreover, to unravel the genetic code of neurotransmitters, are yielding newer strategies in the treatment of neurological and psychiatric disorders.

Not surprisingly, the amygdala contains large numbers of opiate receptors that welcome the brain's own opiates (endorphins) or narcotic drugs. That fits with what psychosurgeons and neurologists have suspected for decades: that this part of the brain is linked to our sense of well-being and pleasure. The thalamus, which carries all kinds of sensory information, including the sensations of touch, pressure, and pain, also has one of the biggest collections of opiate receptors.

The basal ganglia contains many cells that make dopamine, a brain chemical also found abundantly in the frontal lobes that make up the more "emotional" parts of the cerebral cortex. In Parkinson's disease, a disorder characterized by peculiar movements, there is a loss of dopamine in the corpus striatum, a bundle of gray and white tissue right next to the thalamus, and there is evidence to suggest that schizophrenia involves too much dopamine in the frontal lobes. Evidence includes the fact that such drugs (major tranquilizers) that smooth out the schizophrenic's disordered thinking, delusions, and hallucinations block dopamine receptors in the limbic system. These drugs also bind to receptors in the corpus striatum, so that schizophrenics who use the drugs over extended periods of time, may develop a condition known as tardive dyskinesia, a tremor that mimics Parkinson's disease symptoms. And Parkinson's disease patients who are given levodopa (L-Dopa), a form of dopamine, do much better for long periods of time, their tremors and palsy much reduced. But some Parkinson's patients report heightened emotional sensitivity and response.

When early psychosurgeons performed frontal lobotomies on schizophrenics, those they helped probably responded to the surgeons' inadvertent damage to widely dispersed dopamine transmission done by passing wires through the frontal lobes. It must be remembered that in those days there were no major tranquilizers and if a schizophrenic patient had been in the hospital continuously for one year, he was likely to stay there for the rest of his life.

For psychosurgeons of the past, of course, biochemistry of the brain was unknown. General geography was all they had to go on both for diagnosing and for treating mental ailments they associated with this or that address in the brain. Today's neurosurgeons clearly have better anatomical and chemical maps, and although they still labor in a lot of uncharted territory, computed tomography (CT), positron emission tomography (PET), and magnetic resonance imaging (MRI) scanners; brain X rays; and electrical probes guide them away from doing unnecessary damage. Modern neurosurgeons use their relatively detailed knowledge of the limbic system to treat a variety of psychiatric illnesses, and other disorders that have psychiatric components. Because crude maps were all the original psychosurgeons had, the operations they performed were necessarily crude as a result. Among them:

Prefrontal Lobotomy or Leukotomy. Cuts or lesions made into the central core of white matter in the frontal lobes of the brain. At first with injections of alcohol and later with special instruments such as the leukotome ("white matter knife"), Moniz, Lima, Watts, and other early psychosurgeons made patterns of injuries in the frontal lobes to treat schizophrenia, chronic depression, agitation, and just about every major psychiatric illness. Guided only by rudimentary anatomical maps of the brain's major structures and regions, the surgeons reached target tissue by boring through small holes drilled or punched in the skull. In one common operation, they cut two 1.5-inch-long incisions in the skin down to the skull, pulled the skin back with retractors, used a device like an apple corer to penetrate the skull with two holes, about an inch in diameter each, then cut through the very thin meninges or outer elastic layers of the brain's surface and cerebrospinal fluid. The outer gray matter would be divided with a leukotome, before destroying the white matter. The first leukotomes were used by depressing a plunger at one end of a long hollow shaft with a thin stainless steel loop of wire on the other end. After inserting the shaft or cannula into the brain, the surgeon would push the plunger, rotate the instrument, and literally "core" the brain, retracting the loop with as little damage to nearby tissues as his dexterity could manage.

The first patient to have this operation was a middle-aged woman with severe agitation and depression. On November 12, 1935, Moniz's surgeon Lima shaved her head, gave her an enema, and inserted an Avertin suppository to induce anesthesia. He then strapped her to a table and bent her up at the waist on her back with her body at a 45-degree angle to the table. With a sandbag behind her neck to steady and cushion her head, which was bent forward by canvas struts, the brain fibers just behind her forehead were destroyed. After the operation, the woman was reported as being less agitated, but more apathetic.

Standard Prefrontal Lobotomy. This version of the Moniz operation first performed by Lima was further developed and advanced in the United States principally by Freeman and Watts. Using a blunt knife they swept across brain tissue through a temporal or side burr hole on each side of the head, more to the front for personality and emotional disorders and a little toward the back for schizophrenia.

Bimedial Leukotomy. Developed by Milton Greenblott, Harry Solomon, and others at Boston Psychopathic Hospital in the early 1950s, this procedure was a refinement of basic leukotomy designed to limit further the damage to nontargeted brain areas and to limit the desired lesion to the lower-middle quarter of the frontal lobe.

Ice-Pick Surgery, Transorbital Leukotomy, or the Poor Man's Lobotomy. In the search for an operation that would result in less personality damage, surgeons knew they needed to avoid mutilating so much of the frontal cortex white matter to reach the critical parts of the frontal lobe connected with the thalamus. Freeman principally, but other U.S. surgeons as well, first adapted the work of an Italian surgeon, Amarro Fiamberti, who perforated the skull by going through the eye sockets, or orbital plate of the skull, then dividing sections at the base of the frontal lobes by pushing the Moniz leukotome into the puncture holes.

However, this instrument could snag and pull at brain tissue and blood vessels. It took a long time and a full hospital setup. So Freeman in the 1940s tried a variety of instruments on cadavers and settled on a version of an ordinary ice pick taken from his kitchen drawer and later modified.

As noted earlier, the first patient treated by Freeman, secretly in his office, was a woman named Ellen in January 1946, after unconsciousness was induced by electroshocks. Pulling back the upper eyelid, the surgeon placed the sharp tip of the pick into the tear duct. "A light tap with a hammer," he wrote in one description, "is usually all that is needed to drive the point through the orbital plate."

Because this operation required no stitches or conventional anesthesia, nonsurgeons performed it, much to the dismay of neurosurgeons. Thousands of these operations were performed in secret and in state mental hospitals. But the poor and abandoned were joined by thousands of upper-class patients in private sanitoria and clinics, whose families "volunteered" them for the procedure. Freeman developed later versions of ice-pick surgery using a thicker instrument to probe 3.5 inches into the brain.

One of his most famous patients was the actress and star Frances Farmer, a rebellious hellion whose behavior often is compared to Jane Fonda's during the Vietnam War protests. Both shared a penchant for political activism and were accused by some of having communist sympathies. In his chilling biography of Farmer, *Shadowland*, William Arnold described her at age 34 as having "one of the strangest psychiatric case histories on record." Labeled a woman with a lifelong impulse to resistance to authority, she wound up in Western State Hospital where she got insulin shock, electroshock, and experimental drugs to treat a variety of bizarre symptoms throughout the 1940s. Freeman was by then claiming that his ice-pick surgery was as simple to use against psychotic misfits as penicillin against bacterial infections, and he prescribed it for radicals, homosexuals, and other "deviants."

Here is how Arnold described Farmer's surgery:

> The tormented actress was held before him. He put electrodes to her temples and gave her electroshock until she passed out. Then he lifted her left eyelid and plunged the icepick shaped instrument under her eyeball and into her brain. [After doing a number of other patients, Freeman left. William Keller, superintendent of the hospital, walked out sickened.] ... An hour later, Keller returned to the operating theater and found everyone gone. He walked into the anteroom and looked at the postoperative patients resting on cots. One woman was silently weeping and several others were staring blankly at the ceiling. Near one end of the row of patients was Frances Farmer. She was, for all purposes, ready to be released. She would no longer exhibit the restless, impatient mind and the erratic creative impulses of a difficult and complex artist. She would no longer resist authority or provoke controversy. She would no longer be a threat to anyone.

The vivacious and beautiful actress ended her working days as a clerk in a San Francisco hotel and died of cancer in 1970, never heard from again on or off a stage.

Given the complexities of the limbic system, those who pioneered psychosurgery are an appropriate subject of awe. Some were brave; others, swollen with bravado. Both characteristics rocketed them to great heights, drove them to great depths, and left us with twin legacies of shame and hope.

CHAPTER THREE

THE LEGACY OF LOBOTOMY

What nature does blindly, slowly and ruthlessly, many may do providently, quickly and kindly.

—SIR FRANCIS GALTON

Lobotomy and its facsimiles were destined to fall out of favor and ultimately out of use. Expectations trumpeted by psychosurgery's advocates were too inflated not to burst. The *New York Times* in an October 1949 article, for example, wrote that "surgeons now think no more of operations on the brain than they do of removing an appendix."

The problem, of course, was that the operations went too far and too fast and the bad outcomes outdistanced both successes and the capacity of the medical profession to separate what worked from what didn't and good candidates from bad ones. Compounding the situation was the almost total absence of governmental, medical, and legal regulations to control the abuses that came with the medical profession's status and the arrogant disdain triggered by any attempt to question the appropriateness of the operations. Among the worst of the consequences were the suppression of scientific method and scientific lessons and the loss of whatever predictable benefit there was for patients, physicians, and mind-brain research.

In all the feverish activity of lobotomy's Golden Age, nowhere was there a resolution of the basic conflict: Were any of these treatments useful and should they be encouraged; or should we shore up every crack in the dam that buried them, with the conviction that humans have no business messing with the mind?

Historically, medical treatments and operations that boom so rapidly bomb badly when their popularity outruns their proven value; they become the targets of intensive criticism in and out of the medical community. Coronary bypass surgery and heart transplants are two recent examples. With psychosurgery, increasing reports of abuses, failures, and long-term results that were nothing to brag about both fed and ensured the backlash. The operation's appeal could not outstrip its critics forever. Slowly, through the 1950s, psychiatrists, surgeons, hospital administrators, and patients' families began to acknowledge that the intellectual and social limitations of patients after psychosurgery kept most of those operated on in institutions or at least in supervised care.

Walter Freeman did his last transorbital lobotomy in 1967 at Herrick Memorial Hospital in Berkeley, which lifted his surgical privileges after the patient, a woman, died. California by then had become almost the last refuge of psychosurgery's scoundrels. Universal revulsion was setting in against all physical therapies, including insulin and electric shock, for mental illness and by 1970, only 300 to 400 operations were reported nationwide, most using the new stereotactic frames and pinpoint targeting of brain tissue. Neuroscientists were demanding funding for treatment alternatives, including new drugs. (Smith Kline and French brought the first major tranquilizer, Thorazine, to market in 1953.) And protests over the whole idea of tampering permanently with the mind, led by whistle blowers, the counterculture, and civil rights activists, finally buried wholesale classical psychosurgery, driving its preeminent practitioners out or underground.

That might seem the end of the story, a simple case of obsolescence and curious aberration. On the contrary, however, the fall of psychosurgery, like its rise, is a far more complicated tale. And far more instructive.

For one thing, the story isn't over. Just as classical psychosurgery waned, brain scientists began, in fact, to demonstrate that some of the scientific ideas behind lobotomies were valid. New information fueled new kinds of surgery for psychiatric disorders, many now still done in the United States and abroad, and there is renewed interest in the subject among medical experts and patients. For another, psychosurgery's shortcomings were ignored by laymen and scientists alike for decades, too long to accept its prevalence and endurance as an "aberration." The "better mousetrap" explanation for the demise of psychosurgery doesn't fly well, either. Psychosurgery had *not* proven ineffective, and as University of California, San Diego, sociologist Andrew Scull put it, "psychosurgery was never tried on its merits."

Controversy alone didn't kill it, either. Psychiatry had already begun to abandon psychosurgery in the mid-1950s, long before the counterculture politicized psychiatry in the 1960s and 1970s. "In this sense," writes one historian, Harvey Simmons, "the public controversy surrounding lobotomy was a case of driving a nail into an already sealed coffin."

For all these reasons, understanding the last days and the legacy of classical psychosurgery has importance and urgency. Too much has been forgotten, or never learned, about pyschosurgery's Golden Age. Much can be gained by examining its origins, exhuming its skeletons, and analyzing the wounds that killed it.

Its most prominent skeleton is psychiatry's rank abuse of authority. "Psychiatrists did in fact abuse their authority by administering psychosurgery in a broadcast and careless fashion," writes Simmons. He goes on:

> From the mid-1940s to the late 1960s, decisions about lobotomies, about who was to have them, how they were to be done, whether or not there were to be statistical studies of the patients and whether the policy was to continue were made by the narrow circle of medical doctors and bureaucrats which [already controlled the medical and psychiatric establishment].... Whenever an outside influence threatened to impinge on policy, the wagons were drawn into a circle and attackers fended off.... In some cases, psychosurgery was administered to ease staffing problems, for experimental purposes, or simply out of sheer curiosity.

Actually, Freeman and James Watts did report their failures—almost boasting about them, in fact, as a cynical means of justifying quick applications of new "refinements." As one contemporary put it, "failures were merely bumps along a road to glory." They openly acknowledged that 20 percent of their first 500 cases were total failures, but considered that an acceptable record. Nor were they much distressed at the intellectual damage they caused. "It is better for [a patient] to have a simplified intellect capable of elementary acts," they wrote, "than an intellect where there reigns disorder of subtle synthesis. Society can accommodate itself to the most humble laborer, but it justifiably distrusts the mad thinker." Selecting candidates for lobotomy and criteria for performing the operations were developed without much consideration for human rights and were justified with exhaustive, seat-of-the-pants, make-it-up-as-you-go-along accounts of "before and after" symptoms.

William H. Sweet, a neurosurgeon at Massachusetts General Hospital who championed psychosurgery through the 1970s, admits that in the early days of the standard lobotomy, only one prospectively controlled trial—the gold standard of experimental medicine and surgery—was done, and the results were hardly an unqualified success. The study was done in six Veterans Administration hospitals on 373 patients from 1950 to 1952, of whom 140 were operated on and the rest were unoperated-on controls. All but 12 were schizophrenics, considered the toughest and least responsive to psychosurgery. In eleven of thirteen factors evaluated, the 140 operated-on patients all had better mental health after the operation than before: less restlessness, less paranoia, less depression, less anxiety, fewer hallucinations, less anger, and so on.

But by year four after surgery, that translated into fewer than 20 percent who actually went home, compared with 10 percent of the unoperated-on patients. And although 23 percent of the 26 who got radical lobotomy went home, their adjustment to the outside world was "below average to marginal." The study's follow-up did not take into account the fact that advent of drug treatments by the late 1950s meant that both lobotomized and non-lobotomized controls out of the hospital were getting medications, making comparisons of the two groups impossible.

Nevertheless, Sweet has argued, this "carefully designed and executed" study proved that "thoughtful, conscientious psychiatrists in the forties and early fifties had sound reasons for recommending as many lobotomies as they did." And in truth, few let any facts get in the way of progress. Psychosurgeons pressed on, doing lobotomies for schizophrenia, melancholia, mania, anxiety, compulsive behavior, hostility, hyperactive behavior in children, and pain. A steady stream of articles about the occasional dazzling successes lured poor and wealthy families of even minimally sick people (mostly women) to seek lobotomy to cure them of whatever anybody thought was unpleasant behavior.

As for the lobotomists, they reported their results in language that today is shockingly racist, sexist, and unscientific. Freeman and Watts, for example, noted that women did better after surgery than men because they were "protected" at home; that highly educated patients did better than the intellectually less gifted. Black women did better than white women, while Jews had the highest successes because of "greater family solidarity manifested by these people."

When the house of Moniz finally came down, participants and nonparticipants, like field and armchair generals in every campaign, weighed in with interpretations of events and lessons. Many are in print. Others were solicited for this account. Their opinions are strong. Their verdicts are in.

High among the forces they say accounted for the actions of those who embraced and later abandoned psychosurgery were compassion, training, changing circumstances, and economics.

"I was completely turned off by Freeman's ice-pick surgeries," acknowledges Boston neurosurgeon H. Thomas Ballantine. "But when I opened my practice, I did a lot of disc surgery (for back pain) and realized the very close relationship between pain and depression. Treatment of pain wiped out a lot of depression, and psychosurgery seemed reasonable." Tens of thousands of return-ing World War II veterans—suffering both wound-inflicted pain and the depression and self-destructiveness of what we now know as posttraumatic stress syndrome—were frequent candidates for lobotomy, Ballantine adds. At least one study comparing rates of discharge in VA hospitals found that 60 percent of operated men got some benefit. "The critics of psychosurgery often ignore the reasons we did these operations."

Oscar Sugar, retired professor of neurosurgery who trained with Freeman and Watts, argues that he—and many surgeons—did leukotomies as part of necessary scientific studies to compare their effectiveness with equally upsetting treatments, including electroshock and carbon dioxide inhalation. And once the results showed that psychosurgery was not a panacea, many medical sci-entists abandoned it.

Louis Jolyn ("Jolly") West, who was head of the California Cen-ter for Reduction of Violence during the Reagan years as governor and has practiced "biological psychiatry" since 1949, is more defensive, and blames the fall on cycles in (usually misguided) public opinion. Many people confused pop culture with science, he says. "In the aftermath of Ken Kesey's *One Flew Over the Cuckoo's Nest,* anyone who was operating on anyone else's pre-cious brain was a Frankenstein. I thought it was a marvelous novel and made a great play and movie but it was not an accurate por-trayal of either ECT or lobotomy."

Noting that Kesey was a drug addict who had worked in a locked ward of a men's mental asylum, West claims that the novel-ist "used what he knew something about" to pillory a society that had disillusioned him and deprived him of his liberty. Amplifying the Kesey message, West says, were the science fiction stories of L. Ron Hubbard, who craftily leveraged his own experiences with psychiatric illness and fear of electroshock therapy into the world-wide business of Dianetics and Scientology, which essentially declares that all psychiatry is an evil plot.

Rather than a backlash, West sees the fall of psychosurgery as a "frontlash," a direct consequence of the same public distrust of institutions that fostered the work of Kesey, Hubbard, Watergate, and Vietnam and threatens innovation today. "The counterculture had an image of repressive society interfering with their right to do their own thing and picked out a number of things it could play on, including somatic treatment of mental illness. It didn't matter if some patients benefited. Those patients had no voice in the counterculture."

Doctors, West says, did not kill psychosurgery or create the demand for it. "It came from where it always comes, the public, because you can't keep knowledge down. People hear about progress and they want it for themselves or their loved ones, then they demand that the profession provide it. That's the whole history of psychiatry and medicine. A few pioneering doctors were willing to stick out their necks on behalf of desperate people. Ordinary people thought lobotomy would help millions and they clamored for it."

If there's a villain in the story, West says it is our national character along with the human condition. Like the doctor in Henrik Ibsen's play *The Enemy of the People*, destroyed for warning his town of a financially desirable development that would poison their water supply, professional warnings of psychosurgical abuse always existed but fell on public as well as professional deaf ears. "In this country, we tend to go too far one way or the other. In the long run, the public calls the shots, but in the short run, the majority is usually wrong, not right."

Social scientists who analyzed the psychosurgery years between 1935 and 1960 say the key lesson to be learned is that surgical advances and competition among doctors—in the absence of all regulation—often overwhelmed society's ability to react quickly to abuses. In the case of psychosurgery, the new technology outpaced their ability to deal with it, much the same as the Nancy Cruzan case showed that intensive care units had outpaced our legal, ethical, and moral responses to hopeless cases.

Compounding the problem, psychosurgery developed at a time

when rigorous evaluation of cases demanded of today's surgeons by journal editors, laws, and government watchdogs was entirely unknown.

"There were so few controls over what went on," says sociologist Scull, "that we don't even have an accurate count of how many had lobotomies. The estimates I've seen range from 50,000 to 150,000 worldwide. No one was compelled to publish anything and there was no standardization, making follow-up essentially useless." The National Institute of Mental Health, between 1949 and 1951, published critiques of the deficiencies of follow-up studies, lack of controls, imprecise criteria for outcome, and the general poor quality of evaluations and reporting in the treatment of all psychiatric disorders by Freeman and his cohort. But it wasn't until 1971 that Freeman published a long-term follow-up of 707 schizophrenics operated on 4 to 30 years earlier. Some 73 percent were still in the hospital or in a "state of idle dependency" at home.

Scull, an expert on the rise of organized psychiatry, suspects that psychosurgery, along with the absolute monopoly that psychiatry seized over the treatment of the mentally ill, was the only means psychiatrists could muster to protect their medical and professional status from the threat that psychology and Freudian thinking posed. Sigmund Freud, says Scull, was a "mixed blessing" for early twentieth-century psychiatrists. Their mainstream medical colleagues, whose peers they considered themselves to be, were hostile to Freud. But the public was mesmerized by Freudian psychology and demanded its perceived benefits.

Psychiatry's response was to welcome the platoons of neurotics who came to them for treatment, but also to look for physical ways of treating them, to keep their credentials high among the mainstream physician community.

"Whenever doctors are threatened by something they can't explain and can't treat—madness, for instance—they tend to regress to organic models, to look for biological causes," Scull says. "Madness needed treatment so it became a medical problem, and soon all the things no one could explain, such as social pathology, criminal activity, and all kinds of nonconforming behaviors, became medical problems too. Even child rearing. Kids didn't behave? Didn't get toilet trained? Call in the doctors. That's how the whole child guidance movement got started in the 1920s."

Superintendents of state mental hospitals, whose institutions had become horrific dumping grounds in the 1920s and 1930s, felt even more left out of mainstream medicine than psychiatrists in private practice. And they latched on to brain surgery as a way back in. Brain surgery was "new and sexy" and could be pioneered without constraint in their hospitals. The grim death and injury rates? No problem. "Remember," Scull notes, "that Harvey Cushing at Hopkins was just inventing modern neurosurgery as a subspecialty for treating brain tumors and his mortality rates were horrendous, too. By analogy, the back wards of mental hospitals were a long horrible death while brain tumors were a quick horrible one, so it was easy to rationalize the bad outcomes of psychosurgery." Scull also explains that

> the rules of surgical innovation are still relatively relaxed. Even now, the idea of controlled trials in surgery is almost anathema among surgeons. It's considered downright unethical. That's the surgical mentality: If you have what you think is a better way to do something, do it, now, to help *this* patient on *this* table. Maybe surgeons need that personality trait, to be aggressive treaters, in order to cope with procedures in which eighty percent will die if you treat and one hundred percent will die if you don't. But there are side effects to this attitude. Ignoring opposition is one.

As early as the 1940s, it was clear there were lots of failures and bad effects of the operations, and in fact, there was a frantic search for safer operations, Scull says. "But for doctors at that time, trying to find an operation designed to damage the brain without really damaging the brain was like trying to find a nonaddicting morphine. It took them time to realize it wouldn't work, and overall, the profession wasn't willing to give up."

The contest between physical and psychological treatments

that brought psychosurgery to the forefront of medical practice today continues, Scull insists, between psychotherapists with medical degrees and others, like social workers and behavioral psychologists, without M.D.'s. He predicts the battle will lead psychiatrists deeper into the use of drugs and surgery in mental illness if for no other reason than to protect their "market share" and limit the appeal of nonmedical practitioners. "We'll see more biologizing of psychiatry," says Scull, "because these are the only exclusive items physicians have to sell." Is that potentially abusive for patients? Perhaps.

Another possible scenario, however, is that psychiatrists may be far more cautious—even to the point of denying drugs or surgery to those who need them—because of the heavy price they are already paying for past excesses. This, too, is a legacy of psychosurgery's decline. In a paper presented in the spring of 1987, historian Simmons argues that the sharp political and legal curtailment of psychiatric authority the world over can be directly linked to the abuses of psychosurgery. "Unquestionably," he writes, "one reason for the restrictions imposed on psychosurgical operations and for the continuing attempts to circumscribe the authority of psychiatrists is the public's belief that psychiatrists have abused their authority."

To other observers, the rise and fall of psychosurgery fits into longtime Western sympathy for equating "feeblemindedness," "bad blood," and mental illness with social deviance, criminal behavior, immorality, and degeneracy. These beliefs, which fostered the notion that the mentally ill were nonetheless responsible for their "shameless" behavior and in need of punishment, also fostered any number of schemes for "purifying" and civilizing society with technical fixes. Among them: the racist-driven eugenics movement, sociobiology, and psychosurgery.

"There is a long U.S. history of punishing the mentally ill and ignoring the civil rights of such people," says Daniel J. Kevlas, author of a detailed history of eugenics and an expert on the social abuse of science. "If people see the mentally ill as defective and

dangerous, something like psychosurgery becomes not only necessary but humane. The elimination of 'inferiors' was an obligation
felt by many well-educated leaders of society, who looked to science and medicine to use their skills for that purpose."

Kevlas argues that "whenever society is stressed people look for
solutions out of what is contemporary and popular." In the early
1900s, millions believed that antisocial behavior was rooted in
mental illness and that epilepsy, criminality, immorality, and insanity were all due to "tainted" genes that could be bred out of society. Coupled with the rise of neurosurgery, the new science of
genetics, Darwin's biology of natural selection and survival of the
fittest, and the psychiatric profession's turmoil, this belief furnished a recipe for psychosurgery.

There was, in summary, an astonishing willingness and desire in
the late nineteenth and early twentieth centuries to look for and
apply technological "fixes" to all social and human problems. And
only when the beliefs that generated the quick fixes proved impo-
tent, or led to outrageous acts (the Holocaust was one) did these
experiments, including psychosurgery, begin to fail.

Kevlas and other historians say it is hard to exaggerate the popularity of such beliefs among the nation's most prominent and
best-educated citizens, including the Rockefellers, Harvard University president Charles Eliot, social reformer Emma Goldman,
and George Bernard Shaw; such famous geneticists as Raymond
Pearl and Herbert Jennings of Johns Hopkins, Clarence C. Little,
J. B. S. Haldane, Julian Huxley, and Thomas Hunt Morgan; and
top professors at Columbia, Cornell, Brown, Wisconsin, North-
western, and Berkeley.

Victorian attitudes and Freudian psychology's emphasis on sexuality and sexual repression as a guiding force of human behavior
also played roles in the rise and fall of psychosurgery. Many
lobotomies, for example, were performed on the institutionalized
mentally ill to stop or limit "bizarre" sexual behavior, which at that
time meant masturbation, homosexuality, and for women, almost
any overt desire for sexual release. Moreover, since the social the-

ories of the time embraced the idea that the mentally ill were also bad people, it followed they should not be able to enjoy themselves sexually or any other way.

In that sense, forced sterilizations and the psychosurgical treatment of "abnormal sexuality" were an almost natural outgrowth of social reformers who sought to forbid supposed sexual excesses in the "inferiors" that they themselves were ambivalent and ashamed about. Certainly, the therapeutic results of such operations can't explain their popularity. One study of fairly modern psychosurgery (stereotactic hypothalamotomy) done on 70 sex offenders and proclaimed "deviants" in West Germany from 1962 to 1975, for instance, investigators found that "indications for surgery [were] based on questionable scientific and clinical grounds and practically [excluded] psychotherapeutic ... aspects."

A clear message out of this history is that an uncritical search for technofixes to social problems at times of social crisis always leads to overconfidence and abuse. Moreover, says Kevlas, "given that changes in individual attitudes inevitably affect ... institutional actions, both public and private, history surely teaches that we should pay serious attention to warnings ... however shrill they may sometimes be."

Then, as to a large extent now, however, the medical profession was not into heeding warnings, shrill or otherwise, or into criticizing colleagues. The social values of the 1940s and 1950s—primitive by today's standards of sensitivity about civil rights, women's rights, legal protection for patients, and bioethics—were dominated by a "let's try it because I say so" authority of the medical profession. In an era unfettered by an aggressive legal fraternity, physicians did what they thought was called for, consulting only the patient's family (if available) before decisions were made.

That professional arrogance was reinforced by what was then—and still is—the strongest measure of "success" in any mental illness therapy: getting a patient out of a hospital and back home. There was little notion of the heavy emphasis we now all place on "realizing individual potential" and "maximizing individual achievement." Thus patients who after lobotomy were still in need of sheltered care at home and "protection" from the complexities of modern life were not considered bad off at all. This was particularly true for women, who before the consumer and feminist movements of the late 1960s and 1970s were still considered the "weaker" sex and "successful" if they could maintain some semblance of a "happy home" à la June Cleaver. It's common to read in clinical reports of those days comments from doctors about a woman's preoperative and postoperative ability to function only as a wife and mother. Britain's Geoffrey Knight, for example, now in his eighties, still shows photos of women he operated on with the comment that after operation they were able to leave the hospital "and make Christmas for their families" or attend "tea parties."

As for attention to human rights in today's terms, mental patients barely counted.

Consider this entry from Freeman and Watts in their textbook:

> [Case 238 was] brought to the George Washington University hospital in shackles by ambulance from the Midwest where he had been a difficult patient for eight years. He had a fiery red beard and red hair, and one leg amputated at midthigh. He was cursing so loudly and waving his stump so violently that the special nurse who was waiting to go on duty refused to take the case and the superintendent of the hospital refused to admit the patient. We were unable to persuade them to change their minds, so ... the patient was transferred immediately to the psychopathic unit at the Gallinger Municipal Hospital and then to St. Elizabeth's Hospital where we performed a lobotomy in May, 1944. The patient went back to work part time in September and has continued to be more or less usefully occupied....
>
> Other patients can't be dragged into the hospital and have to be held down on a bed in a hotel room until sufficient shock treatment can be given to render them manageable.... Some patients come to operation at the end of a long and exasperating series of medical treatments, hospital treatments, shock treatments, including endocrines and vitamins mixed with their physiotherapy and psychotherapy. They are still desperate and will go to any length to get rid of their distress.... We like both of these types. It is the fishy handed, droopy faced individual who grunts an un-huh and goes along with the family when they take him to the hospital that causes us to shake our heads and wonder just how far

we will get. [But] the [cooperative] type of patient ... makes an excellent witness during the ordeal of prefrontal lobotomy.

If there is a common thread in all of these lessons and legacies it is that psychosurgery's historic excesses and abuses were not an aberration but in fact were far scarier for being right in the mainstream of medical, psychiatric, and social thinking. When the current shifted, psychosurgery was swept away.

A second thread is that there *were* successes. Not all was gloom and doom. A review of 415 schizophrenics by Sweet found that of patients whose psychosurgery was done before a year's hospitalization was ended 57 percent had jobs or were keeping house compared with half that percentage in those who were operated on later in their illnesses. Half of depressives and 75 percent of OCD patients appeared to benefit in numerous reviews, including independent psychiatric evaluation of Knight's British patients. But dredging information out of case documents proved so subjective that even today, scientists seem unwilling even to try.

In the end, the experts conclude, psychosurgery fell in on its own failures, like some power drunk giant who collapses carelessly on his own unsheathed sword. After decades and tens of thousands of patients, the poor results for so many patients simply became too much to ignore. By 1960, even those who argued for less destructive, more controlled operations in smaller numbers of patients had lost most of their support and the patience of the medical establishment, and none too soon to satisfy the growing chorus of criticism. Said Sweet in what was essentially a delayed obituary in 1973,

> The unfavorable features of follow-up observations, combined with the advent of whole families of valuable psychotropic drugs and electroconvulsive shock therapy, led to a massive reduction in the use of neurosurgical therapy. One evidence of this was the huge hiatus in international psychosurgical congresses after the first one in Lisbon in 1948. Mainly in Great Britain, a steady evaluation by psychiatrists of surgery for psychiatric disorders continued throughout the fifties, the

operations usually being limited to the medial or to the lower quadrants of the anterior frontal white matter. . . . Gradually in the sixties, cerebral surgery for psychosis was ... much less wholesale [in] fashion.

If there was a final push off the edge of world medical practice, it came from the creep of new science. At the time Antonio Egas Moniz first learned of Becky and Lucy, scientists already were contradicting the notion that the brain's functional sites operated in an isolated way and were publishing evidence that the brain contained delicate feedback systems in its wiring that integrated emotion and memory, learning and behavior, and primitive and higher-level functioning.

The vehement criticism that came along just kept driving the same nails into the already sealed coffin. But it did further damage. Oregon and California outlawed the practice of psychosurgery—Oregon in 1973 and California three years later—and at the turn of the last decade, other states also were considering such legislation. The backlash also forged strategic partnerships in and out of government to help pass and enforce strict regulation of psychiatric institutions, sometimes impossible informed consent laws, and supreme mistrust of somatic therapies.

Psychiatrist Melvin Sabshin, one of the great "establishment" psychiatrists, has done some heavy thinking about the excesses of his profession over the past 40 years and notes that once "desperate measures" are used in medicine—not just in psychiatry—they tend to become institutionalized and overused. Psychiatric institutions were desperate; they sheltered an environment, a population, and a professionally overburdened staff that nurtured the thought of a quick fix. In the absence of outside brakes, psychosurgery got out of hand. And so could it and other treatments once more.

Psychosurgery's halcyon days produced some new knowledge, and triggered perhaps more medical, ethical, moral, and social conflict than any other form of drug, surgical, or psychological treatment in history. Today, psychosurgeries like those performed in that era are so despised it's hard to find a popular reference to its founder, Egas Moniz—there is none in the *Encyclopaedia Britannica*, for example, or the new *Random House Dictionary*. Try looking up "lobotomy" in any home reference, almanac, or even textbook in psychiatry or psychology. Citations are scarcer than hen's teeth.

Nevertheless, the final legacy of psychosurgery's original promise is that it moved a hardy corps of physicians, surgeons, and advocates for the mentally ill to persist—*very* quietly and *very* selectively—with modifications of psychosurgery that did more good and very little, if any, damage.

CHAPTER FOUR

LESS OF THE KNIFE: THE NEW PSYCHOSURGERY

I had this flea planted in my ear about using less of the knife, which could only mean finding a way of creating a very minute lesion in the brain without destroying tissue on the way in.

—GEOFFREY CURETON KNIGHT, *M.D., FRCS, FRCPSYCH.*

The drive through old residential neighborhoods of southwest London ends at a paved circular drive bordered with shade trees and gardens, their roses in bloom, and a deep lawn that stretches back to the road, sheltering the old buildings from the noise of traffic. Patients and staff of the Priory Hospital go and come through the administration wing at the center of the drive, and its lobby, more like a drawing room, with upholstered furniture, 20-foot ceilings, and uncurtained bay windows. Up a steep flight of stairs to the rounded waiting room and office suites, tea comes in china cups and the carpets are Oriental, and there, chief psychiatrist Desmond Kelly holds up X rays to the light in front of a balcony window.

"This is Susan," he says in a soft voice. "I first saw her in this very room just a few months ago. Let me tell you about her."

While much of the world medical community trampled each other in the 1960s' rush to abandon psychosurgery, a small group of neurosurgeons, psychiatrists and neurologists, particularly in the United Kingdom, stood their ground. "Britain continued with psychosurgery during all the time it dropped out of favor in the United States," according to Kelly. "There was never a stampede in or out of it." His own, and his colleagues', quiet defiance of popular opinion is responsible for Susan's story.

An American now in her twenties, Susan was diagnosed with classic, chronic obsessive-compulsive disorder (OCD) five years ago. Eventually, almost completely disabled by the relentless course of her disease, her psychiatrist recommended inpatient psychotherapy at a famed psychiatric clinic. She would need at least 18 months of hospitalization, her psychiatrist said, during which more drugs and behavioral therapy might stop the endless rituals that were destroying her life and her desire to live. There were no guarantees. The proposed hospitalization was the last straw for her boyfriend, an Ivy League–trained lawyer, and in early 1990, he sent Kelly a letter.

With passion and pain, he entreated Kelly and his surgical colleagues at Priory, to operate on Susan: "I have had the previous misfortune to be with Susan through much of her ordeal," he wrote.

> I've seen the total emotional devastation of this disorder at the clos-est possible range without having it myself; I've witnessed her growing sense of hopelessness as each new wonder drug has utterly failed to achieve any significant suppression of her OCD. I've seen months and years of fruitless psychotherapy and watched her endure the agony ... and anxiety ... of behavioral techniques at the hands of very gifted therapists, only to be crushed once more by the realization that their ministrations, while helpful to some, are not for Susan. I can tell you, Dr. Kelly, that without the surgery ... Susan will die [by suicide]. There is simply no way to live with the demons of OCD.

Moved by the letter, and aware that, indeed, the risk of suicide in the 20 percent of long-term OCD patients who are drug resis-tant, is close to one in six, Kelly accepted Susan as a patient.

By the time Kelly showed her X rays to this writer, Susan had undergone a limbic leukotomy, and was back in the United States in the postoperative care of doctors at a university medical center in the southeast. Her recovery has been excellent. A report from her doctor in late 1991, said "she continues to maintain her level of improvement, which has a course of behavior therapy and is on 50mg of Anafranil.... Her only residual symptoms are occasionally doing brief rituals like wiping off the doorknobs and telephones." She, too, has written to Kelly, to say how unfair it is for people to have the catastrophic illness that she has had and not have faster, easier access to the operation her exceptional resources helped her find an ocean away.

Susan is among hundreds, perhaps thousands worldwide, whose OCD has been brought under control with an operation that severs nerve connections in the brain's cingulum and lower midquarter, an operation similar to the subcaudate tractotomy developed by Geoffrey Knight. In one group of 148 patients rated six weeks and 20 months after surgery at Priory's psychosurgical unit, 84 percent of OCD cases showed significant improvement.

At Massachusetts General Hospital in Boston, a team led by neurosurgeons H. Thomas Ballantine and Robert L. Martuza, and psychiatrist Michael A. Jenike report equally good results on patients with OCD who underwent stereotactic cingulotomy. In a 1987 report on 198 patients with OCD followed an average of eight and a half years, for example, they say 13 percent are fully recovered; 23 percent, functioning normally with some medication; 51 percent, better but with some degree of psychiatric disability; and only 12 percent, unchanged or worse off. That's a "got better" rate, Ballantine says, of 60 to 80 percent. In another series of 696 cingulotomies, Ballantine notes only two cases of paralysis or seizures, testimony to the safety of the operations. The suicide rates for both the British and U.S. OCD patients after surgery is about 5 percent, compared with 15 percent for unoperated-on patients.

Cingulotomies and related operations have helped hundreds of psychiatric patients with other psychiatric symptoms as well. At Brook Hospital's Geoffrey Knight Center in southeast London, a group now headed by psychiatrist Paul Bridges has performed nearly 1,200 stereotactic subcaudate tractotomies over the past 25 years. The 90-minute operation, pioneered by the neurosurgeon for whom the unit is named, uses radioactive yttrium introduced on small ceramic rods into the brain. It has produced 60 to 80 percent success rates against severe depressive psychosis, intractable anxiety, phobias, and panic attacks—as well as OCD—with only a single death and a 1.5 percent postoperative rate of seizures. At Atkinson Morley Hospital in London, limbic leukotomy, a very different operation, has helped 80 percent of patients with obsessive compulsive disorder, 60 percent of chronically anxious, depressed patients, and 41 percent of a mixed group of 17 patients with anorexia nervosa, personality disorders, intractable pain, and obsessive language disorders brought on by Giles de la Tourette's disease (an inherited disease marked by physical and mental tics). Other teams of psychiatrists and neurosurgeons have begun to explore the use of psychosurgery in panic disorders and chronic pain syndromes that produce psychoses and behaviors associated with pain. In the United States and abroad, surgeons now very rarely do amygdalotomies to control for violent behavior caused by brain damage, and occasional reports have suggested benefits from neurosurgical operations for inherited and acquired forms of self-injurious behavior syndrome associated with suicidal depression and drug addiction.

Increasingly detailed knowledge of the three-pound adult human brain makes all of the target areas of psychosurgery more accessible, and good outcomes possible with far less damage to tissue, between the surface of the brain and the target site. These days, for example, surgeons and psychiatrists are careful to conserve and protect the brain's principle parts—the cerebral cortex and the brain stem. The brain stem, often called the "smell," "old," or "primitive" brain because it has been around in mammals the longest, rests in the lower center of the brain, nearest the spine, and in fact, connects the lower brain to the spinal cord and the rest of the peripheral nervous system. The brain stem runs the

autonomic nervous system (involved in such "involuntary" or auto-
matic activities as heartbeat and heart rate, breathing, swallowing,
sweating, and coughing) but is also the "junction" of connections
and paths for senses and movement orders to and from the brain,
muscles, and joints. The autonomic nervous system consists of two
parts: the sympathetic nervous system, which uses energy to speed
up the pulse and tense involuntary muscles, and the parasympa-
thetic nervous system, which calms everything down and saves
energy. The autonomic nervous system is, therefore, vital in regulating emotional and metabolic reactions to fear, anger, joy, and
sexual arousal.

Medical scientists work even more carefully around the cerebral cortex, the familiar pink-tinged "gray matter" that covers the
two equal hemispheres of the brain. Making up the cortex is a
one-eighth-inch-thick canopy of nerve cells (gray matter) that is
wrapped around the so-called white matter, a different group of
cells that guide impulses in an orderly way, like traffic signals
route cars, along nervous system pathways. The cerebral cortex is
the most highly evolved part of the brain, the part that defines
most of what we value as human characteristics of rational thought
and creativity. All of our voluntary movements—those we consciously decide to initiate—begin in the cerebral cortex, along
with our senses of sight, sound, smell, touch, and feel. The cortex
dominates thinking, language, speech, and some parts of memory
and emotion, and it encloses and protects the ventricles, four hollow cavities in the brain containing a cushion of cerebrospinal
fluid.

All information coming into the brain from the peripheral nervous system—nerves that reach from the brain and spinal cord to
the rest of the body carrying sensory information and directing
muscles to move—is handled by large parts of the cortex divided
among the lobes of the brain's two hemispheres. The parietal lobe,
for instance, located at the top of the brain, handles leg and arm
movement. Other lobes include the occipital, at the back of the
brain, which handle vision; the temporal lobes, located above the

ears on the sides, which control memory, speech, and hearing, among other things; and the psychosurgeon's earliest target, the frontal lobes, implicated in memory, learning, IQ, emotions, and in a broad way what we call personality or temperament.

Perhaps the tenderest attention goes to the largest part of the cerebral cortex, running from behind the forehead to the center of the brain. These frontal lobes are responsible for conceptual thinking, for recruiting information from all parts of the brain's memory banks, and for judging and planning behavior. Rear portions of the frontal lobes are also involved in voluntary movement of our limbs and body.

When neurosurgeons-in-training hold a brain in their hands, today they have in their heads fine mental maps obtained with CT scans and other X rays. They know the precise location of the cerebellum, or so-called small brain. About the size of a peach, it has its very own grooves and hemispheres and its duties are control of "fine" motor activities and coordination of muscles. A good cerebellum lets us pick up a needle or a baseball bat with just the right amount of grip, pressure, and control; to hold an egg as safely as a bag of groceries.

And neurosurgeons understand intimately the "operating system" or "logic"—the software—that operates the cerebral cortex. In fact, there are two systems.

The first imposes "sidedness," or what scientists call contralateral control, rules that give the right side of the brain control of the left side of the body and vice versa. The second imposes specialization and localization, via cellular and electrical connections that link particular functions of the brain—sometimes directly and sometimes in a very roundabout fashion—to particular locations or clusters of cells in the cortex. And all of these connections "talk" electrochemically back and forth with other parts of the brain and central nervous system.

Scientists today are mapping the cerebral cortex, preparing detailed guides to mind-brain locations. The geography is complicated and no individual "home" addresses are yet known, much less rooms in those houses. But they have identified details of some metropolitan areas and even some neighborhoods. For example, the visual cortex is at the back of the brain and completely separate clusters of cells have been discovered by PET and MRI scanners to be responsible for what our brains do differently when we see a word, as contrasted with when we hear or speak the very same word. The brain's main speech and language center, directing the formation of words and sounds, is on the left side in the temporal lobe, a part of the brain called Broca's area.

With all this knowledge, surgeons and psychiatrists still do not precisely know how and why psychosurgical operations work, but they are not "experimenting" on the brain or taking random potshots. Enormous progress has been made in developing standard operations and reaffirming the value of psychosurgery in the treatment of resistant emotional and mental disorders.

Today, as Knight explains, there is "far less of the knife," and far more to the science and predictable results for hundreds of patients a year in Britain, the United States, Australia, Canada, Europe, and South America.

For that, they can thank pioneers like Knight, whose career spanned the bad old days of the lobotomy and helped drive the search for less damaging procedures.

Fans of mystery novelist P. D. James will quickly recognize the Camden Hill, west end London neighborhood where Geoffrey Cureton Knight, at 84, and his wife, Bet, still live in a 250-year-old house filled with antiques, photos of their children, and an overlarge dog named Sam. Knight (finally too crippled with pernicious anemia, retired a decade ago) clearly recalls the great pioneers of psychosurgery. His development of stereotactic subcaudate tractotomy—still used today—puts him among them.

On a warm, fall day in 1990, nattily jacketed in a navy blue blazer ("It's 30 years old"), he meticulously reviewed more than 50 years of psychosurgery with a trace of bitterness for the present "underground" state of his craft. His message was clear: Psychosurgery developed—at least in most hands—with great regard for scientific principle, respect for human values, and a desire to do less and less damage in the course of repairing the mind. Among his prized possessions is a letter received in 1964, after delivering the Hunterian Lecture at the Royal College of Surgeons. ("I wore this very blazer that day.") Sent by the great anatomist Sir Wilfrid le Gros Clark, who trained Knight at Barts College, it said, in part: "I feel sure you must feel great satisfaction in turning misery into happiness in so many cases." Later, standing ramrod straight without his cane in front of an ornate silver service presented by the family of Egypt's King Farouk ("I operated on his niece"), he filleted and carved luncheon's salmon with surgical grace.

Knight's first exposure to psychosurgery occurred 65 years ago, when he was a 19-year-old student. He recalls:

> I heard a lecture by a very famous professor of anatomy at Barts. In a cast-off remark, he said the lower part of the brain's frontal lobe contained the tract of emotional expression. That fascinated me, to know that an anatomical tract could have a functional significance of that sort. He went on to say that the lower, inner part of the frontal lobe contained fibers going down into the internal capsule [of the lobe], which were connected to parts of the brain stem having to do with phonation. That's the way we vocalize, by opening and closing muscles involved in speech. My teacher also said these same fibers were concerned with facial expression. And it struck me right then that these fibers were quite obviously pathways of outward emotional expression.

Knight followed up his interest, without much success at that time. "I looked and looked and looked and there was nothing published on this. It was a throwaway remark, as I said, and I couldn't find any literature to support it. But I kept in my mind the thought that if these fibers were the pathway of emotional expression, they must be related somehow to ... how we act out emotions." By that time, Knight knew he would pursue a career in neurosurgery and he began to mature in his chosen specialty just as Egas Moniz came on the scene:

> His contribution to all this, of course, was the injection of alcohol into the frontal lobes which produced a flattening of emotion and a degree of tranquility. This discovery was followed by the destructive operation of leukotomy (lobotomy) in which the whole of the frontal lobe was cut across ... in an effort to divide unknown nerve pathways serving abnormal expressions of emotion while leaving normal emotions intact. And it didn't succeed. It produced a serious flattening of emotions, the so-called frontal lobotomy syndrome, by willy-nilly destroying those pathways. Plus, it inflicted severe damage on other pathways in the frontal lobe. Yes, one got from this operation a degree of tranquility in some subjects, but what you also got was a diminished capacity for the enjoyment of work or leisure. This was a very serious complication because it limited a patient's rehabilitation. Some people also developed epilepsy or suffered paralysis due to division of important nerves. As you know, I'm sure, the whole venture gradually led to resentment and lack of confidence in the whole principle.

Sharing that lack of confidence, as did most of his peers in the field, Knight was by then an assistant surgeon in neurosurgery at West End Hospital and was invited in 1942 by Rolf Strom-Olsen (an eminent British psychiatrist) to join up with him at the Runwell Hospital in Essex. That hospital was a Royal Society research center and Strom-Olsen was going to study the effects of lesions at different parts of the frontal lobe on patients with depression, agitation, violent aggression, destructive behavior, and the like.

> It seems I was still guided by my childhood interest in tracts of emotional expression. It occurred to me that what good there was coming from any lesions was in the lower inner part of the frontal lobe, so I started off by modifying Moniz's original cut—which went right across the whole lobe to produce an effect on the emotional circuits. I was looking for a way to keep the good effects, without damaging the core of white matter and other areas well away from where we wanted to be. I decided that part of the problem was the way the instrument was inserted into the frontal lobe.

In what was to become the first of many modifications, Knight created an operation in which he approached the target in the limbic system from the temple side. "I exposed the lower part of the lobe and put a leukotome in horizontally. I moved the instrument downward just until I felt resistance, then swept it laterally, or to the side. That was the first lower-segment leukotomy."

"The results," he says, "were much better than the Moniz operation because it avoided damage in important areas we knew could not be involved in modification of the emotions.... Soon, the workload increased not only at Runwell, but also in other hospitals in that area. I did altogether about 400 of these modified leukotomies. Some of the results were quite brilliant, and I was satisfied that we were on the right course by trying to divide only the lower, inner fibers with a limited incision. But the results were often far from what we wanted."

There was an initial ten years of excitement about the restricted leukotomy. Then, psychiatrists turned against it because it was quite obvious that the undesirable effects of these gross lesions still far outweighed the benefits. Fibers were cut that involved not only emotional activity but also intelligence and drive. "We helped people with the worst of their symptoms, but certain patients couldn't lead a normal life and didn't enjoy any improvement you might have produced. Some became childish in their behavior, retarded, euphoric, irritable," Knight said.

After World War II, there was a scramble to get out of leukotomy altogether and replace it with localized lesions on cortical areas. Wilder, Penfield and others were highly successful using much more localized lesions in the cortex in a few patients. They had fewer undesirable side effects. This was valuable information because it showed that the real target to aim for was not the central core of white matter but only the cortical areas directly concerned in emotional activity. (In 1948, Penfield, a neurosurgeon at Montreal Neurological Institute, published results of an operation he called a gyrectomy, in which he cut out very selected pieces of the cerebral cortex of the frontal lobes. Ironically, Penfield did not consider his operation very good and he abandoned it.)

It turned out that the areas Penfield hit on were in the cingulum portion of the frontal lobes and in the amygdaloid nucleus in the temporal lobe. These areas appeared to be too far apart to be influenced surgically by a single cortical lesion.

"But here is where I was very lucky and I do mean lucky in what happened next," Knight recounted.

> Things had happened which led me to produce a single lesion that did interrupt the nerve fibers from *both* of these areas at a point of *convergence* without destroying the cortical areas involved. How this lucky thing came about is interesting. It started initially from work [William] Scoville did in the U.S. around 1950. [A Hartford, Connecticut, surgeon, Scoville developed an "open" operation, slicing down the front of the scalp to the eyebrow, to destroy frontal lobe tissue just behind and above the area of the eyeball. He called it "orbital undercutting" and the direct visualization his open wound permitted let surgeons aim their knives more selectively.] The result was to make an opening in the dura and separate the target cortical areas from the underlying white matter. Scoville had devised methods of undercutting each of the cortical areas important in psychiatric patients, including the cingulate gyrus and the orbital cortex. Sometimes he would isolate fibers on the inner site of the lobes and sometimes the orbital. The best results, in my opinion, were obtained by undercutting of the orbital cortex, but it appeared that we didn't need to isolate the whole orbital cortex by an undercut that went right across the lobe. Too much damage there and in the wrong place.

It struck Knight that because these cortical operations worked, there *had to be* nerve fibers converging from these areas on to the orbital cortex. Otherwise how could he explain Scoville's success? What's more, these fibers also had to lead to the subcaudate area, where fibers not only ascend to the cortex but also return from down there, creeping under the head of the caudate nucleus to affect the hypothalamus and brainstem areas. "Okay, I thought, well, right, all we need to do is to confine our cut to a narrow strip, perhaps two centimeters wide at most and coming in under the head of the caudate nucleus and interrupting fibers from the cingulum, amygdala, and orbital areas where they come together."

Knight designed such an operation, calling it restricted orbital undercutting. Just cutting a narrow strip, going down under the head of the caudate nucleus to a point a good six centimeters from the tip of the frontal lobe. The good results were unexpectedly successful to a lot of people, because previous work had suggested such an incision could bring disastrous results if the downward, descending cut hit the corpus striatum. Knight didn't let that happen.

First of all, it turned out that the fibers in the cingulate area descended right into areas 13 and 14 in the back, or posterior, segment of the frontal lobe from which fibers appeared to relay signals onto the hypothalamus. So he and other surgeons were really getting their effect in a sort of roundabout way without damaging the head of the caudate nucleus.

They also learned that multiple combined lesions produced entirely different effects from the single lesions. In studies in cats, for instance, "you might get tranquility from one lesion but if you damaged an adjacent area you might get aggressiveness or violent behavior," Knight said.

> Finally, we found out that our new operation put the lesion directly over areas 13 and 14 of the orbital aspect of the lobe, so you had a lesion affecting fibers from the cingulum coming down and from area 13 coming up to duck over into the hypothalamus. Most remarkably, there were also fibers from the amygdaloid region coming up into the rear part of the area where we made our lesion, fibers that sort of turned over and nicely descended into the hypothalamus too. We were getting three lesions for the price of one cut. And they were not antagonistic. Instead, they combined to produce a beneficial effect. But the best part was that papers were describing circuits coming out from the hippocampus and thalamus, which we already knew were important in maintaining normal emotional activity and this lesion I made was below them and didn't affect them at all!
>
> Here we were right in the clockworks of a point of concentration, convergence really, of fibers from all the primitive parts of the cortex which had come down into this area very obligingly just awaiting our single lesion. I just couldn't believe the luck! But that's what we stumbled on.

Knight's "luck," of course, was based on more than a decade of hard work and observation. But he also reports an almost transcendental vision that advised him to "go further back and use less of the knife," to go further back, that is, in the frontal lobe, which would involve areas that could not be approached from above, but only horizontally. Early leukotomy lesions had shown that vertical cuts to this area produced very damaging results.

But Knight had observed that in cases of previous failed leukotomy, the restricted orbital undercutting encountered the old vertical scar at about four centimeters from the frontal pole. This was cut through and the incision continued for another two centimeters over the rear orbital cortex. The results were remarkable. What all this meant was the target area should be a zone having length and breadth, but little depth.

Less of the knife also meant less damaging instruments, such as stereotactic devices and other means of making precise lesions without destroying tissue on the way to the target area. "My search for less of the knife," he recalls, "was then rapidly accelerated by very good hearing on my part."

Smiling, Knight recalled how he overheard a young surgeon who had been listening to his lecture saying that *he* was going to organize a stereotactic operation in that area of the brain and decided that he himself had better get moving. He sought help from colleagues in the Department of Medical Physics at the Royal Postgraduate Medical School who were dealing with radioactive isotopes packaged in radioactive seeds. They told him that they could indeed produce very controlled localized lesions using the seeds. A professor in the department worked out the precise mathematics of the dosage in order to supply the necessary radiation and distribution of effect with the seeds. The recommendation was to plant four rows of two seeds, each row on either side of the target area. To do this, Knight modified a stereotactic device adding a needle carrier that could be moved to the four sites for implantation, as well as an implanting needle adjustable for depth.

The results showed a remarkable change in the patient's emotional behavior and no harmful effect on intellect or personality. The results were particularly beneficial in elderly patients who suffered severely from the depressive illnesses of old age. Thus was born in 1971, the modern bifrontal stereotactic tractotomy. The first operations were performed at the Royal Postgraduate Medical School, but later, when stereotactic facilities were provided, at the Regional Centre at the Brook Hospital, where they named the psychosurgical unit after the man who developed the new procedure.

By the time Knight retired, in additional to a full load of standard neurosurgical procedures in a busy unit, he had personally performed 400 cases of lower segment leukotomy, more than 600 cases of restricted orbital undercutting, and more than 1,200 cases of radioactive stereotactic tractotomy, some 2,200 procedures in all. A few stand out in his memory. "I remember Bessie Garrod. She was the worst case I saw in my career. She was 79, bedridden, with a sixteen-year history of severe melancholia. She just lay in bed, muttering and chewing her lips into massive granulations. No drugs helped her. We inserted seeds, and after bilateral implantation, she blossomed like a rose. In three months time, she was animated. At six months, she was attending tea parties. For me, that's what this was all about."

"The results of today's operations, those developed by people like Knight, can only be called impressive in properly selected patients," says Kelly.

> And if we didn't wait years and years to consider the surgery, until patterns of behavior associated with the illness were so rock hard and intractable and the patients so frustrated and demoralized, we would do even better, in my opinion. People can come too late. I've had people kill themselves between the referral to our unit and the time of their appointment for evaluation. If you have people who are so deteriorated that they've lost all support systems, all hope, you won't get as good results.

It's time to get beyound the emotional baggage of the past and systematically study the possibilities for even more kinds of psychosurgery. Progress in understanding the emotional brain and its connections already have proven that cuts or lesions in nerve pathways between the frontal cortex and limbic system's deep structures can help a variety of psychotic and psychoneurotic illnesses. Surgical risk has been greatly reduced with stereotactic techniques, in which precise advance measurements in three-dimensional space guide surgeons safely to specific brain areas. Using a small radiopaque frame attached to the head, and X rays and radiation-sensitive electrode tips, surgeons can get to targets a millimeter in diameter in the cingulum, amygdala, hypothalamus, stria terminalus, and hypothalamus. And quantum leaps in diagnosing brain disease, understanding brain chemistry, mapping the brain with precision, and cloning genes that make chemicals that control thought and feeling could yield new operations, as well as new drugs for mental illness.

"We threw the baby out with the bath water once and shouldn't do it again," says Colorado psychiatrist Clyde Stanfield. "I was witness to the bad times, but there is a role for psychosurgery." Drugs may have revolutionized the care of the mentally ill, and reduced the demand for "extreme remedies," but sentencing someone to life in chemical or physical restraints also demands a responsible look at alternatives.

New forms of psychosurgery are such an alternative, and some psychiatrists are increasingly unwilling to deny them to patients and their families because of past history. And they chafe at what they consider a conspiracy of silence from medical scientists and hospitals. "The message for patients and their families," says neurosurgeon Ballantine "is that surgical help is available, safe, and effective, but if you want it and need it, you must ask for it. What could turn everything around in the U.S., what is slowly turning it around, I think, is that there are more psychiatrists who are biologically and physiologically oriented and genuinely looking for ways to help desperate patients."

The desperate are legion.

A report released in the fall of 1990 by the Public Citizens

Health Research Group and the National Alliance for the Mentally Ill concludes there is a "near total breakdown in public psychiatric services in the United States." The survey notes that:

- There are more than twice as many people with schizophrenia and manic-depressive psychosis living in public shelters and on the streets (at least 150,000) than there are in public mental hospitals.

- There are more people with schizophrenia and manic-depressive psychosis in prisons and jails (about 100,000) than in public mental hospitals.

- Increasing episodes of violence by seriously mentally ill individuals are a consequence of not receiving treatment.

- Mental health professionals have abandoned the public sector and patients with serious mental illness.

- Frustration and anger also are building among Americans as they see their neighborhoods and downtown areas blighted by those who cannot care for themselves, and their taxes skyrocketing to pay for more welfare and psychiatric services. Experts estimate that 30 percent of the 500,000 homeless in the United States suffer from manic depression and schizophrenia, along with 10 percent of those in jails. The Los Angeles County jail alone reportedly has 3,600 psychotic inmates and uncounted others live in U.S. versions of Third World slums. According to Lewis Judd, M.D., former director of the National Institute of Mental Health, only 1 in 5 of the 2.8 million Americans with serious mental illness receive adequate (not state of the art) care. Because AIDS, dementia, and the aging of the baby boom generation are likely to swell the number of older mentally ill in the next decade, 70 percent of our mental health care dollars will probably go for episodic, nondefinitive, revolving-door hospital care. The federal budget for mental health research, moreover, at $515 million in 1990, is a fraction of the billions spent on cancer, AIDS, and heart disease research.

Psychosurgery cannot correct those numbers, but its new versions of operations that influence emotion and behavior can be part of the solution to intractable mental illness. Controls that protect patients from freewheeling surgeons and psychiatric abuse are firmly in place, making the new psychosurgery safer and undermining arguments that the operations are abusive. Permanent, yes. Unsuccessful, sometimes. But abusive? No more—and usually less—than most neurosurgical procedures.

For example, the Cingulotomy Assessment Committee at Massachusetts General Hospital withholds surgery until two neurosurgeons, three psychiatrists (one of whom, Edwin Cassen, is also a Jesuit priest), a neurologist, a nurse, and outside psychiatric counsel agree it's needed. The referring psychiatrist must provide follow-up care after surgery. "We may decide the patient is not a candidate, that the patient might be but has not exhausted nonsurgical treatments, or that the patient is a candidate," Ballantine says. If the committee decides the patient is a candidate, members still interview the patient in person to see if paper indications match the personal, more subjective indications. Only then is surgery is scheduled. "We don't operate on patients who can't or won't give consent, and who have no surrogate to stand up for them."

Growing confidence in the operations has tempered precautions with a commitment to helping patients faster. In Britain, Kelly says, "we have safeguards, but we don't sit on cases for months and months. We give patients a decision, one way or the other, in a few weeks at most." There is evidence, moreover, that the "watchdogs" are more and more willing to bow to psychiatric and medical judgment when cases are close calls. Kelly tells the story of a very depressed woman turned down by the Mental

Health Commission for psychosurgery. "We had strongly recommended surgery. They said no. She tried to hang herself. Then the council reversed their decision. She's been working for the United Nations since her surgery, and I think lessons were learned all around." The commission serves the purpose of preempting emotional debates about psychosurgery, but clinicians are in charge of the decision making in most cases.

Despite lingering political and legal concerns, success after success is building fans for the new psychosurgery among doctors and patients, and expanding the definition of psychosurgery to cover operations not principally designed to alter mood or behavior, but which have that effect anyway. For example, operations that interrupt nerve pathways to control pain or disabling movements frequently also modify depression, anxiety, and other psychiatric symptoms. Disconnecting pain nerve pathways in the brain to stop terminal cancer pain or the vicious facial pain of trigeminal neuralgia has been found to eliminate the profound, drug-resistant depression and anxiety its victims develop over years of suffering. More than 500 operations—many in China and South America— have been done to implant active brain tissue into the brains of Parkinson's disease patients in an effort to control their jerky, disabling movements. These operations may be honestly described as a form of *psycho* surgery, given the behavioral as well as physical problems associated with the disorder and the remote likelihood that the operations will reverse or cure the disease.

In addition to *cutting out* a problem area of the brain, the new psychosurgery may also *add* material to replace, repair, strengthen, or restore a missing or malfunctioning part of the mind with brain tissue implants, the introduction of new genes into the brain chemical factories in the central nervous system, or insertion of synthetic versions of chemicals that manipulate and control mood and thought. Specialists now believe that surgical lesions in the brain help patients not only by severing faulty circuits but also by producing secondary biochemical changes in the naturally occurring forms of these chemicals and by making the brain more sensitive to helpful drugs. Other parts of the brain may also make more chemicals. "The brain is always trying to maintain a state of equilibrium," explains Kelly, "and this may well account for the phase-in course that recovery takes following psychosurgery, during which time chemical balances are restored."

Under these terms, candidates for "psychosurgery" might include patients with overactive thyroids, overactive sex drives, drug addiction, schizophrenia, traumatic brain injury, learning disabilities, migraines, alcoholism, hormonally linked disorders such as premenstrual syndrome, and pedophilia. Many, if not most, neurosurgeons will object to such a list. At Johns Hopkins, for example, a prominent surgeon told me that "in my opinion, none of these are appropriate candidates for psychosurgery." Still, the potential for such expansion is there—for better or worse—and the list could include not hundreds of people but many thousands.

It's possible, perhaps probable, that drugs and preventive measures will eventually do away with the need for all surgery for mental illness, much as oncologists plan for the day when surgery for cancer will yield to drugs; prevention; and less traumatic, risky, or socially undesirable treatments.

Until then, psychosurgery is here to stay. As the operations have moved to smaller, less damaging lesions, "less of the knife"; as new diagnostic and brain mapping capabilities have put precision into the operating field; as side effects have dwindled, disappeared, or become acceptable in number and severity; and as risks have dropped lower than the risk of suicide or total disability in chronic psychiatric patients, psychosurgery has pushed its way back from oblivion.

There is still a need for vigilance, caution, and checks to prevent abuse of patients. But while the scientific, technical, legal, and social issues remain, surgery for the treatment of psychiatric disorders is here to stay and possibly to help more patients with more illnesses.

Here are some of the operations being performed in the United States and elsewhere today, along with the disorders they treat.

STEREOTACTIC CINGULOTOMY FOR
OBSESSIVE-COMPULSIVE DISORDER

Everyone is "obsessive" or "compulsive" to some degree about something. But for those with severe OCD, the hourly and daily rituals consume their lives, disabling them beyond their control. Psychiatrists note that three-fourths of all patients with OCD respond fairly well to behavior therapy and such drugs as clomipramine, fluoxetine, or fluvoxamine. But for an estimated one to two in five patients, conventional treatments do not work. Cingulotomy and limbic leukotomy (see below) offer excellent results with relatively minor side effects, and in 1988, the *Journal of Clinical Psychiatry* carried an article recommending the operation for drug-resistant patients. In general, cingulotomies are lesions in the cingulum placed usually with hot-tipped probes or freezing agents.

At Massachusetts General Hospital, cingulotomy begins with the drilling of two small openings, or burr holes, in the skull through which long tubes are threaded, guided by special X rays called fluoroscopy. Through the tubes, surgeons place a needle that is entirely insulated except for the center of the tip and a little place at the top to which an electrode can be attached.

They then make a ventriculogram, an X ray that uses air blown into the ventricles (or cavities) of the brain to produce a distinctive pattern of shadows. This outlines a piece of the cingulum called the cingulate bundle that is the target of the surgery. The needle is then carefully positioned between the front and back and sides of the target, ready to make two lesions or scars about one centimeter in diameter and two centimeters deep, one below the other, interrupting the circuits that run through the cingulum. The lesions are made by sending a precisely controlled radio frequency current through the attached electrode to heat the tip of the insulated needle to about 80°C for 100 seconds.

Psychiatrists point out that the results of cingulotomy and all psychosurgery could be biased because anything offered as a treatment of "last resort" can be a powerful motivator for claiming success. For that reason, the criteria used for evaluating patients are conservative, but even with the most conservative assessment, 40 to 50 percent of all patients believe they have benefited, and overall improvement has been demonstrated for 60 to 80 percent.

Jenike says a review of the last 25 years' experience with cingulotomy has convinced him that at the very least, 40 percent of the most hopeless patients were helped. "Because it's still hard for us to know exactly why or how the procedure has helped, I had not been an advocate in the past, but after doing this review, it's hard to dismiss it."

STEREOTACTIC LIMBIC LEUKOTOMY FOR OBSESSIVE-COMPULSIVE DISORDER

An operation of choice in the United Kingdom, the limbic leukotomy is similar to subcaudate tractotomy (see below) but is more extensive. It combines lesions on both sides of the cingulum with lesions in the lower front areas of the frontal lobe of the cortex, where many nerve fiber bundles converge as they narrow and pass below the head of the caudate nucleus en route to the hypothalamus and other limbic brain connections. This so-called frontocaudate-thalamic tract appears to carry a network of signals, sometimes referred to as the Papez circuit, which appear to be the key signals in OCD. Some surgeons claim a success rate as high as 89 percent for even the worst patients, a rate better than that claimed for cingulotomy. At the Priory Hospital in London, surgeons often "convert" a cingulotomy into a limbic leukotomy in patients whose OCD persists.

Performed under general anesthesia, the limbic leukotomy takes advantage of X rays, MRI, and CT scans to guide the placement of lesions in the brain. At Priory, the operating-room team first uses electrical stimulation to trigger certain physiological responses that tell the surgeon he or she is aiming at the right spot. The permanent lesions are made through the stereotactic frame. "We were interested in function more than in anatomical sites, so stimulating the target sites would not only give us an important preoperative landmark, but also a way to check results physiologically after surgery," says Kelly.

Kelly used a polygraph, or "lie detector" apparatus, in the operating room to get the tracings while the patient was under general anesthesia. "To our joy, even asleep, we saw clear differences in breathing, heart rate, blood pressure, and blood flow through muscles when we stimulated different areas of the brain," he said. "The best physiological landmark was respiration. The differences were often dramatic."

"What we have learned and been able to track," Kelly explains, "is that there are pathways going from the frontal lobe into the limbic system of the brain where there are two major limbic circuits. One is the defense reaction circuit and the other is the Papez circuit." The Papez circuit runs through the cingulate gyrus. The defense reaction circuit is involved in flight-or-fight responses. But the Papez circuit goes all the way around into the hippocampus, which is in the temporal lobe.

Earlier efforts to interfere with the Papez circuit divided the pathways between frontal lobe and both circuits, a case of overkill. The Freeman-Watts operation divided as much white matter as possible, a frontal lobotomy. Moreover, OCD patients did not do very well after lobotomy. Thus, in 1969, Kelly and a team at St. George's Hospital were asked to devise an operation for OCD patients who failed after a full range of antidepressants, tranquilizers, and clomipramine. The challenge was to make the occasionally successful older operations safer and more predictably beneficial. Published cases led Kelly to suspect that the best results were coming out of operations that somehow reached into the lower quadrant and the cingulate gyrus, but the lesions were too big and too mutilating.

A transfer to the Atkinson Morley Hospital provided the next advance. "They had a stereotactic apparatus, so we could get away from a freehand operation in which a surgeon would literally put his finger in the ear and position his wires into the brain by feeling his way around," Kelly says. "The old operation gave us a target within a centimeter and what we needed was accuracy within a millimeter, an order of magnitude better. The stereotactic frame gave us a way of making a lesion with minimum damage on the way in from the skull."

With the help of his physiological tracings, Kelly and his team also found similar landmarks in both the frontal lobe and the cingulate gyrus. "This was very interesting because these sites are a mile away from each other. If you look at an anatomy of the brain, the frontal lobe and cingulate gyrus don't seem connected in any way, but it meant we could cut less and get results that were at least as good and maybe better." The tracking also demonstrated that the circuits ran to and from the hypothalamus as well, the site of the defense reaction. Stimulating these areas drove the patients' heart rate up from 94 to 140 beats per minute and constricted blood vessels, the same changes that occur naturally when people are frightened.

What gratifies Kelly especially about the high success rate in OCD is that OCD patients are the "least suggestible" and, therefore, the least likely to report success if they did not actually feel greatly improved. "If anything, they are impervious to suggestion," he says. "That's the whole problem." Moreover, Eschsler Adult Intelligence Scale tests given to his OCD and other patients demonstrate that IQ is not damaged by the operation.

STEREOTACTIC CINGULOTOMY FOR DEPRESSION, BIPOLAR DISORDER, AND SCHIZOID-TYPE ILLNESSES

Ballantine recently reviewed 198 patients with depression, bipolar disorder, and schizoid illness on whom he performed stereotactic cingulotomy with an average follow-up of 8.6 years. He reports that 13 percent fully recovered, 23 percent needed medication but were functioning normally, 51 percent had various degrees of psychiatric disability, 17 percent were only slightly improved, 6 percent were unchanged, and 6 percent got worse due to surgical complications or progression of their disease despite surgery and other treatments; 9 percent died by suicide later.

In a series of 696 cingulotomies, there were only two cases of paralysis from surgery and a 1 percent rate of seizures, all controlled by drugs.

STEREOTACTIC LIMBIC LEUKOTOMY FOR ANXIETY, DEPRESSION, AND OTHER SEVERE DISORDERS

Stereotactic limbic leukotomy, which builds on the subcaudate tractotomy developed by Knight, also helps many patients with severe anxiety, depression, manic-depressive psychosis, and related psychiatric disorders.

In one of Kelly's series of patients, 49 were OCD patients, 27 were operated on for chronic anxiety, 36 had severe depression, and 19 showed depression combined with schizophrenia anxiety and obsessive behavior. Patients had been sick anywhere from 3 to 35 years. All but a few of the men had been forced to stop working or take a demoted position, and a majority of the women were unable to run their homes or care for families. Each had an average of four hospital admissions and 69 had made at least one serious suicide attempt. All but 23 had received electroconvulsive therapy (ECT), and 33 of them received more than 50 courses of ECT along with tranquilizers and antidepressants. Results showed that schizophrenics don't respond well and it is a mistake to raise their hopes. But for the rest, using a five-point scale of improvement or nonimprovement, the results showed that at least 40 to 50 percent got better in each category.

STEREOTACTIC SUBCAUDATE TRACTOTOMY FOR BIPOLAR AFFECTIVE (MANIC-DEPRESSIVE) PSYCHOSIS

Psychiatrists L. M. Lovett and D. M. Shaw of the University of Wales College of Medicine, in a 1987 report in the *British Journal of Psychiatry*, described nine patients who underwent subcaudate tractotomy for bipolar disease after all drug treatments with lithium and other medications failed. A majority reported reduced frequency and severity of both "highs" and "lows." Perhaps just as important, drugs that had been ineffective in the past sometimes worked after surgery, apparently making the brain more sensitive to the chemicals. All nine patients had been incapacitated before surgery and radioactive seeds were used to make the lesions.

A second round of nine patients was reported on in 1988 by British psychiatrist Bridges and coworkers at Guys and Brook General hospitals in London. Two to four years after surgery, five showed "substantial improvement" and four had improved somewhat. "These preliminary results suggest that there is a place for this operation in the management of severe bipolar affective disorders which are not responding to any other treatment," the team said, "although decisive recovery occurs less often than with unipolar depression."

STEREOTACTIC SUBCAUDATE TRACTOTOMY FOR UNIPOLAR DEPRESSION

In patients with severe, long-term depression, against which shock treatment and drugs fail to work, the results of stereotactic subcaudate tractotomy have been astonishingly good. In one review of 250 cases between 1972 and 1984, published in 1988 with a minimum four-year follow-up of cases, psychosurgeon Dr. J. R. Bartlett of Brook General and psychiatrists A. S. Hale and Bridges evaluated patients according to the size of their lesions. In all cases, radioactive yttrium rods were placed on both sides of the caudate nucleus to make the lesions, but the size of the lesions— i.e., the number of rods placed in the brain—increased between 1972 and 1984. Those doing the evaluations were not told ahead of time which patients had which size lesions. Of the 250 patients, 170 were female with an average age of 51 and 80 were male, average age 59.2. The patients ranged in age from 20 to 78.

Results: Among the men, a total of 32 patients either became free of depression or substantially improved enough to carry out normal lives. Another 22 improved somewhat but were still considered ill, and 26 either did not improve or got worse. One puzzling outcome: Most of the patients did best with only 12 rods implanted or with 20; far fewer did well with 16 rods—unaccountably. Among the women, 68 of them were in the symptom-free or essentially cured category, 51 improved somewhat, and 51 did not improve or got worse. For them, the more rods, the better.

In two previous studies reported in 1971 and 1975, between 49 and 58 percent were in the most improved or cured categories compared with 40 percent in the most recent study. In the somewhat improved category, the figures were 23, 25, and 29 percent respectively, and in the worst or least improvement categories, the figures were 27, 17, and 30 percent, respectively.

The team concluded that the return to a normal social life after surgery for depression contained important gender differences, and it was harder to assess outcomes for men because of generally high unemployment in Britain and their generally older age at the time of operation. It is easier to assess a woman's ability to care for home and family as evidence of reduced depression.

STEREOTACTIC AMYGDALOTOMY FOR VIOLENCE AND AGGRESSIVE BEHAVIOR

Amygdalotomies directly target the defense reaction circuits that run through the amygdala deep in the limbic brain. Patients are often victims of epilepsy or brain damage that produces unpredictable, uncontrollable rages.

The lesions are made with heat or freezing agents only after electrical stimulation conclusively demonstrates that the rages and violent outburst can be triggered when particular areas of the amygdala or the circuits that lead to them are hit.

Decreases in aggressiveness and other abnormal behavior have been seen in dozens of patients. A typical case was described in 1970 by Vernon Mark and Frank Ervin in a textbook:

> Julia was a pleasant, nice-looking, 21-year-old cherubic blonde who developed severe brain damage and epilepsy after mumps encephalitis at age two. Her epilepsy, which began at 10, was marked at first only by lip smacking, staring, chewing and brief unconscious periods, but this would result in panic and mindless running or flight during which she would carry a knife to protect herself because she often wound up, not knowing how she got there, in a dangerous area of town. Her first serious attack on someone occurred in the movies when she felt an attack coming on, and ran outside telling her parents she would meet them there, but a glance in a mirror in the hallway reflected her in her mind's eye as evil and disfigured. At that moment, unhappily, a stranger bumped into her. In a panic, she took the knife and stabbed the girl.

In the hospital, under electrical stimulation of the amygdala, doctors found that when the right amygdala was jolted with a weak current, Julia bared her teeth, grimaced, lost control, and had a seizure, during which she attacked anything or anyone in her way. After an operation to make a lesion in the right amygdala, she had only two mild rage reactions in the first year, none in the second.

STEREOTACTIC HYPOTHALAMOTOMY FOR VIOLENT BEHAVIOR AND SEXUAL DISORDERS

Similar to the amygdalotomy, for stereotactic hypothalamotomy lesions are made in the middle of the hypothalamus, resulting in reports of 95 percent success in stopping violent, aggressive, and restless behavior. This operation has been done mostly in Japan. Side effects such as hyperactivity and lack of bladder control make this a risky procedure, but in severe cases, worth the risk.

Similar operations to reduce sexual drive are perhaps the most controversial use of psychosurgery. Nevertheless, unilateral lesions made in small areas of the hypothalamus and mammillary complex can result in marked reductions in sexual drive and help a few patients whose lives are out of control. An illustrative case, reported in 1977, involved a 29-year-old man sentenced to six years in prison for multiple rapes. Six months after his operation, he said, "I can converse with women, without thinking of sexual intercourse.... I feel considerably safer and freer. I only regret that this approach could not be used much earlier."

Castration to stop rapists and reduce violent behavior is considered by some a form of psychosurgery in that it is designed to stop abnormal behavior. Sex is not a disease, but the expression of it by some people is psychiatrically pathological. "Chemical" castration, using hormone drugs, is not uncommon in the United States. Depo-Provera, for example, is used in conjunction with psychotherapy at the Sexual Disorders Clinic of the Johns Hopkins Hospital to treat pedophiles and rapists.

The links between sexual behavior and brain circuitry are complicated and mostly unknown, but psychiatrists and neurologists have documented some individuals with temporal lobe epilepsy whose seizures result in full orgasmic climax.

LIMBIC LEUKOTOMY FOR TOURETTE'S DISEASE

Giles de la Tourette's disease is a disorder characterized by completely uncontrollable bouts of motor tics, obscene language, and repetition of words spoken by others. A complex biological and psychological disorder, it does not affect the patient's intellectual abilities or general health, and victims have been successful professionals. However, the disease is often socially crippling, because the attacks are usually unpredictable and drugs and therapy cannot always control them.

The most widely accepted theory of the cause of the disease is an abnormality in dopamine receptors of the basal ganglia, causing too much dopamine—an essential neurochemical—to flood central nervous system pathways. Drugs that affect the dopamine feedback system in the brain have proven somewhat helpful by blocking the dopamine receptor areas. But most patients either are not helped enough by the drugs such as Haloperidol and Clonidine, or resist them because of side effects. Poor results with drugs and behavioral therapy have led to increased interest in using surgery to turn off the behaviors by ablating, or knocking out, the offending dopamine-rich areas.

In a 1987 review of 17 cases reported in the surgical literature since 1969, Italian scientists reported that improvement in symptoms occurred in half the cases. There was no improvement in the others and one man developed stuttering, epilepsy, and motor abnormalities. In a psychosocial study done on eight patients, the operations helped four and failed to help three. The operations ranged from stereotactic thalamotomy, to frontal lobotomy, to the old-fashioned ice-pick lobotomy and leukotomy. None of the older operations was done later than 1981.

Analysis showed that in carefully selected patients, using small, localized lesions that avoid extensive damage to the frontal lobe, results may be good enough to warrant offering it to intractable patients. Two patients in Britain who had limbic leukotomy included one with a compulsion to touch the back of his eye. Captive of this "tic," he actually put his finger into the orbit and doctors believe he would eventually have blinded or killed himself without an operation. He is doing well, his mother reports. The second patient has not done well. He still has very destructive urges and, his psychiatrist says, "an uninhabitable flat."

In each case, the surgery was designed only to deal with the compulsive aspects of Tourette's, not the underlying disease or the nondestructive tics. Medication can usually handle the milder, more common tics.

A surgeon in Birmingham, England, is reportedly doing amygdalotomy for Tourette's as well, but not strictly for psychiatric indications. The doctor, Theodore Hitchcock, believes the surgery targets a disease state in the brain and may actually cure the ailment. Other forms of so-called self-injurious behavior that don't respond to behavior or drug therapy might also be helped by limbic leukotomy.

STEREOTACTIC LEUKOTOMY TO TREAT DEPRESSION AND PAIN ASSOCIATED WITH CANCER

Having brain cancer is clearly a reason to be depressed, but in some cases, the depression is not just "garden variety," or a consequence of having the illness, but is pathologic in itself, a consequence of brain damage caused by the tumor. Indeed, cancer specialists all know of tumors, malignant and benign, that have gone undiagnosed for long periods of time because the symptoms patients complain about and show are psychiatric, not physical, in nature. In many such cases, drugs actually improved the depression, further convincing the doctors that the patient's "disease" was cured.

MRI and CT scans have shown that some brain damage caused by tumors can trigger anxiety, depression, and even schizophrenia-like symptoms that are indistinguishable from the real thing and almost completely resistant to drug treatments or psychotherapy. In a few cases, leukotomy has stopped these symptoms even when the underlying cancer itself is inoperable or only partly relieved. In one case reported in the *Journal of Neurology, Neurosurgery, and Psychiatry* in 1984, for example, a 62-year-old housewife who had 30 years earlier been treated with ECT and frontal lobotomy for psychotic depression was found to have a long, slow-growing brain cancer. The psychosurgery had stopped her depression, but not, of course, her cancer.

GAMMA KNIFE CAPSULOTOMY FOR ANXIETY DISORDERS

Using MRI to track, map, and provide direct hits over their targets, surgeons and psychiatrists at the Karolinska Hospital in Stockholm and University Hospital in Uppsala, Sweden, apply gamma-radiation through a stereotactic frame to the white matter in the front part of the brain's internal capsule to interrupt limbic pathways.

In a report in a 1987 issue of the *Journal of Neurology, Neuro-*

surgery, and Psychiatry, this so-called gamma knife was used in eight consecutive patients with severe anxiety disorders. The five women and three men were operated on between 1977 and 1979. Each had been ill an average of 17 years and they ranged in age from 22 to 47. Independent evaluations showed five were satisfactorily improved and two were modestly improved. Results on a second evaluation scale found five in good to fair shape (none excellent or superior) and two, poor after surgery.

The authors, led by Per Mindus, conclude that in five of the seven cases, or 70 percent, outcomes judged satisfactory by the patients and their families were closer to the MRI scan's objective evidence of having hit the target. "Despite the small number of cases," they wrote in a journal report, "a statistically highly significant correlation was obtained between clinical outcome and MRI findings." The results should make future psychosurgeries for this disorder even more precise and outcomes safer and better.

PREFRONTAL SONIC THERAPY

First done in 1954 by Pier Lindstrom, prefrontal sonic therapy involves placement of an ultrasound transducer directly on the covering of the brain through burr holes; the sound beam is aimed with the help of a stereotactic device. White matter is highly sensitive to ultrasound, while the cortex is not. Favorable results have been recorded for the control of severe, chronic pain; panic; depression; and obsessive-compulsive disorder. Side effects—dullness, passivity, and seizures—were transient, contrasted with long-term improvement in 50 percent of psychotics and 75 percent of psychoneurotics in one study of 500 patients.

SURGERY FOR FOCAL EPILEPSY

Because epilepsy has behavioral as well as biological components, a few bold physicians will argue that the increasing amount of surgery being performed to stop seizures—especially in children and individuals whose seizures can mostly be controlled by drugs—can also be viewed as a form of psychosurgery. Most of the practitioners interviewed reject the nomenclature, partly out of fear of raising bad, old specters and partly out of conviction. "To suggest that this kind of surgery is psychosurgery is outrageous," was one of the milder objections to including epilepsy surgery in a discussion of psychosurgery at all. Nevertheless, under an expanded definition of psychosurgery as operations to treat emotional, mental, and behavioral disorders, these surgeries fit the category.

For example, at the Johns Hopkins University Medical Institutions, Washington University School of Medicine and Hospitals, and the University of California Los Angeles Medical Center, computer-assisted neurosurgical procedures have moved from a "last resort" to an instrument of cure and control for many patients who want to ease their lifestyles as much as they want to stop the firestorms in their brain.

Focal epilepsy, seizures that arise and remain in a single focus or area of the brain, afflicts an estimated 360,000 people, who are unresponsive or relatively unresponsive to drug control of their disease. The abnormal electrical activity is born of diseased brain tissue, not psychological illness. However, the enormous behavioral and emotional component of epilepsy and the difficulty of unbundling the psychological from the physical in the behavior of patients blur the distinction.

By removing abnormal areas of the brain—and in the case of a group of two dozen patients at Johns Hopkins with a profound form of epilepsy, half the brain—neurosurgeons can eliminate all or most of the seizures and the risk of further brain and psychosocial damage. The surgery also provides total relief from the need to take antiseizure medications, which carry undesirable side effects and prohibit many epileptics from driving cars, participating in some sports and occupations, and having a full life.

Although many doctors will disagree, an increasing number of patients come to surgery not because their disease is uncontrollable, or because it is life threatening or disabling, but for emotional, psychological, and social reasons. Wendy is a strong case in point. As described by her neurologist, John Freeman, M.D., of Johns Hopkins,

> Wendy had her first complex partial [focal] seizure when she was 13 ... and medication was prescribed. Phenobarbital made her sleepy and Dilantin only slightly reduced the frequency of her seizures, now occurring three to four times a week. Tegretol was added ... however, Wendy's schoolwork began to suffer ... and she became depressed. At 16 she couldn't drive and because of embarrassment she became less social and more isolated.... Despite attempts to adjust medication, [nothing could control] her seizures.... She had been turned down by the colleges of her choice.... She was depressed about the seizures and her future.

After surgery to remove the focal seizure tissue in the front right portion of her temporal lobe, Wendy has had no seizures for five years, has finished her Ph.D. in psychology, and needs no medication. "I only wish that we had done the surgery much earlier. It would have made growing up so much easier," she told Freeman.

To see if surgery will help, neurologists and neurosurgeons first carefully stimulate the brain to test motor and sensory responses and map or pinpoint the areas to be removed or short-circuited. With the help of computers that record brain waves from 16 sites, surgeons find out whether the seizures are coming from the left or right side of the brain. Then, under general anesthesia, they open the skull and place a grid of 48 sensing electrodes, tiny platinum contacts on the tough outer layer of the brain. For the next several days, the patient's brain activity is "watched" electronically and videotaped so that doctors can see the relationship between what the patient is doing—behavior, seizures, grimaces, etc.—and the electrical patterns. By sending electrical stimuli through the sensors to the brain, doctors are also able to map precisely the boundaries of vital areas that control speech and movement of facial muscles, limbs, and so on. If the surgeons can indeed find the focal point of the seizures, and it is in a place that is safe enough to operate on without causing damage to vital brain areas, the patient is returned to the operating room and the tissue removed. Otherwise, the grid is simply removed.

At Washington University, results are typical for the centers that do this procedure. In a series of 100 patients—44 of whom were children under 14 years old, including infants, and on whom medication could not control seizures, some occurring up to 50 times a day—60 percent of those operated on with a focus that was accessible had a good result: That is, seizures either stopped completely or were reduced enough for patients to go to school, go to work, or to be cared for outside of an institution. In the remainder, results were insignificant or ambiguous.

At the Hopkins epilepsy monitoring unit, neurosurgeon Sumio Uematsu, M.D., has been implanting the grids for about five years with more than acceptably good results, he reports. In some individuals, like Matthew, whose story is told in Chapter Eight, epilepsy affects behavior, mood, and other psychological activities. Patients may be normal between seizures or they may have automatism, yell, undress in public, get violent, get headaches, and suffer chronic fatigue and depression.

Uematsu has done epilepsy surgery on over 300 patients since 1970, generally removing a wedge of tissue four to seven centimeters. He has done 80 grid implants in the last few years. Of his cases, including the older ones without benefit of implant grid mapping, 50 percent are seizure-free; 25 percent have had a significant decrease in seizures (from two per week to two per year, typically); and 25 percent are no better, or possibly worse.

"Epilepsy surgery is greatest when applied to children because if you can cure the seizures before they crystallize into an adult lifestyle, you convert the patient from a lifestyle of disability and invalidism and all the behaviors that go with all that to one of accomplishment," says Edward Dodson, M.D., professor of pediatric neurology at Washington University. "It should not be a last resort but a first resort. It is or would be the treatment of choice for easily defined lesions in a single focus. The success rate is 90 percent or better, compared with far lower rates with drugs and behavioral modification."

Dodson says the success of the surgery is not yet widely known or accepted among doctors or patients. "That's sad," he says. "Many children have a high probability of a drug-free, seizure-free life with this surgery. There are an enormous number of under-served and unserved patients out there because of our fear of psy-chosurgery's history and baggage. The medical profession has crippled itself unnecessarily."

NEUROSURGERY FOR GENERALIZED EPILEPSY

At the University of California at Los Angeles (UCLA), sur-geons are doing operations similar to the one described above for focal epilepsy on children with generalized as well as focal seizure and again with excellent results. The surgery sometimes apparent-ly works because generalized seizures can originate in a single focus.

This phenomenon was discovered when neurosurgeons operat-ed on a condition known as Sturge-Weber syndrome, in which there is an overgrowth of blood vessels on the surface of the cor-tex accompanied by generalized seizures. When the vessels (or angioma) were removed, *all* the seizures stopped. Now UCLA has applied the idea to children whose foci can't be found with elec-troencephalogram (EEG).

Hemispherectomy, a procedure developed and abandoned years ago in the United States, then resurrected, improved, and championed by pediatric neurologist Freeman and neurosurgeon Ben Carson, has now been performed on two dozen patients with astonishingly good results.

Jane is a typical case. A bright five-year-old, she fell off a see-saw and had a generalized seizure, which a CT scan showed had emerged from damage in the left hemisphere. Soon the whole right side of her body was affected; she limped on the right leg and had speech problems. Then a viral condition, Rasmussen's aneurysm, was discovered and her parents were told the disease would eventually destroy her brain. She would become retarded and completely handicapped. After suffering literally hundreds of *grand mal* seizures a week, she had half her brain removed.

Today, she has only slight use of her right hand. But her speech and reading are entirely normal; she has had no seizures and is on no drugs; she is in the regular third grade, playing soccer. "Clearly, for Jane," say her doctors, "half a brain is far better than a badly functioning whole brain."

Finally, for some epileptics, surgeons section or sever the corpus callosum, cutting tissue that connects the two hemispheres of the brain to prevent the spread of seizures from one side to the other. There is usually a 50 to 70 percent decrease in the severest, generalized seizures.

In March of 1990, the National Institutes of Health held a consensus development conference on surgery for epilepsy and concluded that 10 to 20 percent of the 150,000 who develop epilepsy each year have medically intractable forms that become chronic and "impair the quality of life for all concerned." Thus, they said, up to 5,000 patients a year may benefit from surgery as a treatment. And, they said, because most surgical patients are adults and have had uncontrolled epilepsy for 10 to 20 years, not enough information is available regarding the effects and possible benefits of earlier surgery at a young age, including better health and quality of life. The consensus was that surgery can and should be considered carefully and in a fully equipped epilepsy center.

"Success," the report concluded, "is measured not only by improvement in seizure frequency and type, but also by improvement in behavior."

Whether or not all of these operations, particularly those for epilepsy, are categorized as psychosurgeries, operations to improve the lot of patients with psychiatric and mental diseases are still relatively infrequent. Indeed, and ironically, the success of modern psychosurgeries had been undermined by a severe drop-off in the number of operations performed world-wide. As Knight put it,

> the law now forbids us to make these lesions without an okay by a psychiatrist, and only about 40 patients a year are done at the Knight unit. My procedure is still alive and kicking but underutilized. The worst of it, for me, is that the biggest drop is among patients who most need our help. They are very sick people. I was very excited at the prospect of using my operation widely to reduce suffering among the bedridden, elderly, and infirm in nursing homes and asylums. The mental hospitals are full of old people for whom we could do so much more. For a while I made a beeline for the elderly. Their normal emotions can be released and they can be returned to full activities. We're not doing that. This saddens me more than you can know.

CHAPTER FIVE

PAIN AND PARKINSON'S DISEASE: EXPANDING DEFINITIONS OF PSYCHOSURGERY

> *If you come to me and say, "Should we be doing psychosurgery?" I'd say, "No, absolutely not." But if you come to me and say, "Are there behavioral conditions we ought to consider modifying with surgery on the brain?" my answer is "yes."*

> —GUY MCKHANN, M.D., JOHNS HOPKINS UNIVERSITY

Euphemisms aside, operations on the brain can influence a variety of neurological, emotional, and behavioral symptoms. Those influences can be accidental or incidental. They can also be strategic—planned offensives on one level with the knowledge that they will influence another. By paying attention to the interlocking psychological and physical aspects of psychosis, aggressive behavior, epilepsy, and other disorders, doctors may find surgical approaches that are better, safer, cheaper, and longer lasting than current treatments.

Several conditions are candidates for these strategies because of the widely diffused networks of tissues, cells, and chemical receptors they involve. If psychosurgery has a bullish future, it will be in this realm. Perhaps the best current example of how such strategies may work—and their implications for surgical treatment of psychiatric symptoms—can be found in the story of Parkinson's disease.

Until recently, Parkinson's disease (PD), marked by tremor and muscle-joint rigidity, was considered exclusively a movement disorder caused by biochemical depletions of dopamine and disturbances of the dopamine receptors in the brain or, more simply, by a breakdown or death of cells that produce dopamine, one of the principal chemicals the brain needs to transmit signals among neurons. Patients develop tremors in the hands and arms, slow speech, a shuffling gait, muscle rigidity, and a "masklike" facial expression.

Since the mid-1960s, neurologists have known that synthetic versions of dopamine—levodopa and carbodopa—can relieve symptoms, although within five years or so, the disease can become resistant. In these resistant patients, neurosurgeons in the past sometimes injected alcohol into the brain, apparently stopping some of the tremors by disabling abnormal nerve signal transmission or, possibly, by changing the ratio of dopamine-rich to dopamine-depleted tissues in the brain. Today, because of the vast knowledge of the "integrated circuitry" between the neocortex and the limbic system, including the thalamus, some aspects of Parkinson's are considered psychiatric, involving mood and personality. "Now we realize that changes in thinking and mood in patients are rather common with Parkinson's disease," says Mahlon DeLong, M.D., whose work at Johns Hopkins showed that changes are most likely tied to the disease's effects on circuits other than the ones linked with movement. Moreover, studies show that patients are depressed or anxious simply because the disease exists, not in the way most people are temporarily upset if they become ill.

With Johns Hopkins neurosurgeon Fred Lenz, M.D., Ph.D., DeLong and others have used pinpoint accurate electrical probes to create minute brain lesions deep in the limbic brain and "turn down" key reactions in the gray matter—the cerebral cortex via the circuits that feed in and out of that matter. The tissue most often targeted is in the thalamus, where damage interrupts circuits that run from the cortex to the basal ganglia. These are the same nerve circuits that regulate body and eye movements, thinking, and mood.

So far, the Hopkins team has discovered five separate circuits and has devised operations that have been compared to precision bombing.

Neurosurgeon Lenz helped develop the procedure, called stereotactic thalamotomy, in the 1980s at the University of Toronto. With the patient awake, he first performs CT scans and inserts tiny electrodes into the skull to highlight which clusters of cells are linked to tremors (they react when stimulated electrically). These operations have been shown to provide long-term relief from parkinsonism in up to 80 percent of the patients operated on. Moreover, with PET and MRI scans of specific neurotransmitters and their cellular receptors, surgeons can look directly at the chemical activity and verify that the lesions have actually influenced the physiological progression of the disease.

Yet the fact that surgery helps patients is only part of the story. More intriguing, perhaps, is the light the success of such operations shed on connections between mind and brain, between biology and psychology, and on treatments that affect both. The brain, for instance, has several dopamine "pathways," including the thalamus, hypothalamus, and other parts of the limbic system. These dopamine-sensitive nerve pathways run from the cerebral cortex to the deeper, older brain tissues—the basal ganglia and thalamus—and back again. Moreover, these nerves involve everything from body and eye motions (the sensory-motor system) to learning and mood. (The activities of these dopamine pathways are not yet completely understood, but they clearly relate to emotions, because blocking dopamine receptors with chemical opposites of dopamine is how several major antischizophrenic drugs work.) Keeping in mind the limbic role of the basal ganglia and the thalamus, Johns Hopkins neurologist DeLong and his colleague, Garrett Alexander, looked for and found (so far) five separate circuits in PD patients that interconnect controls for limb movements, thinking, planning, emotions, urges, and drives.

"We used to think of PD as purely a movement disorder," DeLong has said, "but we now realize that changes in thinking and mood in patients are rather common." Knowledge of the psychiatric as well as the biological symptoms showed them where to look for the key circuits. And they've come to understand that depression, anxiety, and other psychiatric symptoms in PD patients are not simply "exogenous," or related to the fact that illness is upsetting in general. Instead, they realize that whatever is biochemically and organically wrong in the brain is producing *both* the physical (motor) symptoms *and* the psychiatric symptoms. All these observations, together and in turn, gave DeLong and his colleagues clues to what happens to particular nerve cells and in what order when PD develops.

Recently, in studies on monkeys, the Johns Hopkins scientists used a potent chemical poison called MPTP to destroy cells on the circuits they believed to be involved in PD. Results showed that MPTP led to Parkinson-like symptoms in the animals and to increased activity in the basal ganglia and a deeply hidden piece of the thalamus called the subthalamic nucleus. The subthalamic nucleus turned out to be a part of the brain never before suspected of playing a role in PD. MPTP also dampened the activity of circuits reaching all the way up to the cortex, circuits affecting movement, mood, and behavior. DeLong has recently put lesions in the monkeys' substantia nigra, a part of the primitive brain, and literally wiped out Parkinson's disease in his MPTP animal model.

The basal ganglia, part of the more primitive brain located near the brain stem, contain masses that have long been known to play a major role not only in Parkinson's but also in other involuntary movement disorders. Damage to the basal ganglia creates not a lessening of movement but a derangement of it, a wildness, made possible by neural connections to the cortex. According to Haring Nauta, a neurosurgeon at Johns Hopkins, basal ganglia signals flow easily in and out of the limbic system, not just involving movement and motor systems but also sidestream signals. Added to what his colleagues have discovered, he thinks it's reasonable to suggest that the basal ganglia reflect and control a whole range of motor-related activities of the brain, beginning with simple movements and increasing in complexity through more complicated sequences of movements to patterns so complex that they can only be called behaviors.

If that's true, there may be a single disease process affecting different points within one of these levels or tiers of the brain and leading to greatly varied symptoms—from tremors to panic attacks, from mental illness to motor disabilities. Says Nauta:

> Perhaps neurological illnesses which today appear very dissimilar, such as movement disorders and behavior (psychiatric) disorders, may some day be shown to have similar pathological mechanisms. What's remarkable about the anatomy of the brain is that the anatomical systems for sensation and emotion are organized along similar, parallel lines. The behavioral apparatus, the part of the brain that has to do with motivation and behavior, the so-called limbic system, those circuits are very close and parallel to more traditional sensory motor circuits.

As brain specialists move through and around these interlocking systems, more ideas for treating *all* of the symptoms of a disease like Parkinson's emerge. For example, in the spring of 1987, *The New England Journal of Medicine* published a report by Mexico City surgeon Ignacio Madrazo, who described dramatic improvements in the tremors of two PD patients who received transplants of tissues from their own adrenal glands into their brains. More than 500 of these operations have now been done in the United States and elsewhere in attempts to reproduce and study the long-term safety and effects.

Are these "psychosurgeries"? Some would say so, pointing to the mild to moderate improvements in neurological and psychiatric symptoms of many of the patients operated on so far. The dramatic advances first reported by Madrazo and several U.S. academic medical centers have not been repeated, but if further careful studies and refinements prove the operations valuable, opportunities for surgery and implants to treat not only PD, but also disorders with PD-like symptoms, are certain to increase.

Also, if laboratory-grown brain cells ever become available as a result of work by Solomon Snyder and Gabrielle Ronnett (see Chapter Six), the future of this kind of neurosurgery seems limitless.

Other scientists exploiting the brain's overlapping networks are finding similar connections between mind and brain in a condition everyone knows firsthand: pain.

Neuroscientists know that as a symptom, pain involves numerous specific pathways in and out of the brain. Deep organ pain, for example, communicates to the brain via different pathways than the pain of a burn. A headache, a bruise, a bad tooth, a broken bone—in all of these acute, or short-term painful events, a specific nerve path is triggered by infection, injury, tension, disease, or combinations of these factors. Pain can be stopped by eliminating the end target of the nerve pathway (the bad tooth and nerve), by treating the infection with antibiotics, by repairing the bone, by interrupting the pain with electrical stimulation or massage, or by overwhelming the pain with aspirin or morphine.

As pain becomes chronic, however, the effects spread. No longer is the pain merely focused in a defined and limited area, but it is then diffused, recruiting different systems of nerves and chemicals and coping strategies. Chronic pain is associated with depression, anger, fear, and helpless frustration, moods that turn on biological and chemical systems that can worsen the pain. And in turn, these emotions can alter behavior in sometimes profound ways, some obvious, some more subtle. Relief from the pain brings changes equally dynamic. In chronic pain, the pathways involve more interlocking systems, running in and out of the emotional circuitry as well as the designated "pain" paths. "In many cases of pain," says Guy McKhann, director of the Krieger Mind-Brain Institute at Johns Hopkins, "the biological and chemical factors that organize pain and emotions at this level are indistinguishable. They overlap and interact and that gives us a pretty good model of the challenge neurosurgeons and neurologists will face in the future."

For those who doubt that pain has a psychological component, studies have demonstrated that even terminal cancer patients can be trained to stop complaining about pain—and presumably stop feeling so much pain—when their anxiety, stress, and reinforcements (such as attention or sympathy) for complaining are reduced. Since the 1960s, behavioral researchers have been able to show that pain is partly a learned response, therefore governed in part by the mind, and that it is possible to lower the amount of morphine given terminal cancer patients for pain when there is a carefully and humanely used system of rewards to encourage behavior that reduces pain—getting up, interacting with others, eating well—and discourages behavior that exaggerates it, such as complaining, tension, and anger.

In one of the most controversial cases ever publicized, psychologist William H. Redd was asked to treat the constant, loud crying of a terminal cancer patient at a California hospital. Despite round-the-clock caretakers and intravenous morphine, the man's wailing "could be heard six rooms away day and night" disrupting the whole floor and the family's limited supply of patience. Redd studied the behavioral, emotional part of the pain, never denying for a moment that biology was to blame for most of it. But he discovered that the wailing increased dramatically whenever doctors, nurses, or family visited. He initiated a form of behavior modification called "time-out" in which all attention stopped when the man cried, except for routine medical attention. There was no conversation, no sympathy, no anger, no nothing. His therapists also encouraged him to use his wailing energy in other ways, including reading and watching television. After ten days, the crying stopped completely. He ate better, he needed less morphine, and he was more alert and in control. He enjoyed his family's visits and they enjoyed him more, so they stayed longer.

❖ ❖ ❖

Given the interaction of biology and psychology in pain, what's the evidence for the idea that modifying the symptoms of pain coming from one part of the brain can influence activities—including behavior and feelings—in other parts of the brain?

One example with growing use in recent years is called TENS, for transcutaneous electrical nerve stimulation. An electrode planted under the skin but over a part of the brain or central nervous system can be "fired" at will by the patient through a remote-control radio-signal transmitting device to stop the travel of pain signals. The device is especially useful in terminal cancer pain and for severe and chronic back pain. Another example are systems that let patients dose themselves with measured amounts of narcotics at their own pace and in tune with their own needs, without waiting helplessly for a doctor to order the drug or a nurse to deliver it. Surgeons have stopped clinical depression and suicides by cutting pain nerve pathways in victims of trigeminal neuralgia. On the horizon are devices that might be implanted in the brain or along the central nervous system to bring drugs or electrical stimulation automatically and continuously.

Studies of TENS and self-administration of narcotics demonstrate that pain is better controlled, patients complain less, less narcotics are needed, and patients *perceive* that they have less pain even though objective measurements suggest that the amount of pain they have has not changed. One way of interpreting such results is to conclude that patients are giving themselves drugs or stimulating themselves in such a way that the pain cannot get as good a grip. But the results also suggest that when people feel in control of a bad situation like pain, they feel less helpless, less depressed, less anxious, and happier. Are their *moods* in fact producing subtle biochemical or physical changes that assuage the pain?

"You could say either, and I think it's both," says neurologist McKhann. He adds:

> If we put an electrode in the body that a patient can, with a remote control unit, use to stimulate and interrupt nerve signals, what is that

patient able to do? And why will he do it? In my opinion, he's not just using it to eliminate something we objectively label "pain." Pain means something very different to everyone. He will use the implant to help him control his *feelings* of pain and about pain. Another way of putting it is that the patient is unhappy with the feeling. And the fact is, you are modifying that patient's behavior—taking him from unhappy to happy—when you give him the means to interrupt that feeling.

Are such people dosing themselves because they are feeling pain, or because they are feeling depressed and unhappy and anxious? Doctors who want to appear objective say it's because they have pain, but in truth, only the patient himself or herself knows how much pain he or she really feels. The other side of this is emotional. When you relieve pain, or let people relieve it for themselves, the fact is that you are modifying a lot of moods and a lot of behavior, too, from immobility to depression to complaining to anger. What you're doing is modifying behavior and mood through a particular means—pain relief.

In essence, surgeons who produce mood or behavioral "side effects" from pain surgery can also be said to be performing psychosurgery and a few admitted anonymously during interviews for this book that they have sometimes done operations more to get the "side effects," and improve "the quality of life," than to directly influence a disease process itself.

No one is "opposed" to surgery or implants or narcotics for pain relief or other distinctly "organic" symptoms, but they may very well be against all of these to treat mental illness. Yet by at least some measures, that is what they do. At Johns Hopkins, Nauta is using intense streams of precisely targeted X rays as a form of knifeless brain surgery to treat deep-brain tumors. He also cuts neural circuits that create intense, chronic pain, particularly in nerves in the head and face. The work, guided by computer programs and stereotactic devices, allows the radiation beams to converge on a problem area from different angles and hit targets as small as 15 millimeters in diameter. "This isn't exactly the conventional definition of psychosurgery," says Nauta, but advances in related realms are here and more are coming. For example, he says, there could well be neurosurgical delivery of drugs that are safe and effective only at a specific site in the brain or that block or enhance or damage only one or a few subclasses of chemicals critically involved in pain transmission such as bradykinin. Bradykinin is produced by the chemical reactions that occur when blood vessels in damaged tissue break. It appears to be the villain in certain kinds of peripheral pain—sunburn, arthritis, headaches—that don't respond to narcotics. Minuscule amounts can create excruciating agony.

Nauta has done experiments in which he injects an antibradykinin chemical called capsaicin into the spinal canal of rats. Theoretically, a disc saturated with a slow-release form of the chemical could be delivered neurosurgically to other parts of the nervous system, including the brain. Drugs to fight brain cancer already have been implanted this way. In the case of the laboratory rats, the capsaicin makes them incapable of sensing pain with their hind legs, yet the tail and legs are fully functional and mobile. The rat also has total control of its bladder and is "perfectly happy and undistressed," Nauta reports. "But they can walk along a grid that is like walking on a hot asphalt pavement barefoot on a Sunday afternoon in July with their hind legs and not feel anything. But they sure won't put their forefeet down." Nauta sees some version of capsaicin injection or implant surgery as a humane alternative to heavy doses of narcotics or severing major nerves to stop chronic pain.

Understanding the neural networks that snake between higher "cortical" functions and the limbic system will, in the future, mean more use of operations able to affect functions "upstream" and "downstream," McKhann predicts, from very specific neural effects to more global ones.

Another condition ripe for this approach to therapy is memory loss related to Alzheimer's disease and other brain-damaging diseases. Acting on the notion that one might preserve memory or other brain functions by replacing cells that may be dying too fast or in large numbers in Alzheimer's disease (AD) patients, a few surgeons have already proposed plans to transplant brain cells along with nerve growth factor to try to preserve the cells' mass and memory.

Because many psychiatric disorders are characterized in part by disordered memory and learning, what's learned with AD patients may have serious relevance to schizophrenics and other victims of mental disease. Studies on the brains and minds of Alzheimer's patients, who suffer increasingly severe memory loss, suggest that while short-term memory is controlled by fairly well-known areas and systems in the brain, long-term memory activity is really quite global and diffuse throughout the brain. It's conceivable, though pure speculation, that there are regions in the brain that can be stimulated via surgical implants or drugs that would actually improve memory. Would this be an operation to modify behavior? Psychosurgery?

McKhann, among others, bats off the term. "We need to stay away from the old bugaboos." But, yes, he acknowledges, surgical approaches already in place and others on the horizon will capitalize on the brain's complex neural systems to modify emotional and behavioral symptoms.

CHAPTER SIX

FRONTIERS: PSYCHOSURGERY IN THE FUTURE

Man can learn nothing except by going from the known to the unknown.

—CLAUDE BERNARD

One morning in 1987, medical student Jeffrey Nye hurried to an operating room at the Johns Hopkins Hospital with a petri dish full of a sterile culture solution in his hands and stood by as surgeons removed an entire half of a toddler's brain in an effort to save the other half from a deadly and progressive form of epilepsy. Pediatric neurologist John Freeman had invited Nye to the operation, designed to create a neural "firebreak," because he knew of a research project Nye desperately hoped to move forward. The operation ultimately failed; the 18-month-old died. But the gram-size cube of her cerebral cortex that the surgeon deposited in Nye's dish that day lived on, establishing the world's first living culture of apparently normal human brain cells.

Nye's mentor, Solomon H. Snyder, M.D., is a psychiatrist and director of neuroscience at Hopkins. For years, he and his colleagues had tried with frustrating lack of success to grow normal, human brain cells in the laboratory. A human's brain cells, trillions of them, are all present at or soon after birth. Unlike other cells in the body, they neither divide nor multiply and without that arithmetic, the effects of damage, disease, or missing cells are permanent. Although drugs and surgery can repair or overcome some ill effects, neuroscientists have long sought a way to repopulate or reconstitute brain cells. The first step is to grow and study them.

Snyder, Nye, and principal research partner, Gabriele Ronnett knew that hemispherectomy patients' brain cells were—biochemically and anatomically—nearly indistinguishable from normal neurons. What was wrong were the connections, the wiring, the transmission signals between them. The cells fired too often and at the wrong times, resulting in dozens, sometimes hundreds, of crippling *grand mal* seizures a day. They also knew from their colleagues in pediatric neurology and surgery that the surviving halves of the brains after surgery in the youngest children were exceptionally "plastic," able to take over many of the jobs of the lost hemispheres and restore the children to near-normal lives. Johns Hopkins has in fact won a worldwide reputation for the operation and annually hosts an energetic reunion for children once consigned to institutions and early death. These kids now have brains that work very well, indeed.

But beyond the clinical advantage, Snyder and Nye saw something else. Were there, he wondered, some characteristics of these very young children's neurons—their youth, their plasticity, their sensitivity—that might get them growing and dividing in his test tubes and give science a normal, or essentially normal, brain cell population? Nye's mission that day in the operating room was to retrieve the surgically removed hemisphere quickly and give the scientists a chance to find out.

Two years later, in March 1990, the journal *Science* published the news that the Johns Hopkins team had become the first to grow and maintain a continuous test tube "line" of apparently normal, living human brain cells. Cancerous brain cells had already been grown because one of the earmarks of cancer is perpetual growth. But cancer cells do not have normal biochemistry or genetics and are, therefore, of limited value as models for studying normal brain activity or as potential sources of treatment.

As the story broke around the world, Snyder and Ronnett explained that the cell culture was an important step in growing enough human cells consistently over time to study their natural patterns, their biochemistry, and their function. These cells could be manipulated to mimic and thus become models for serious brain-related illness, from Parkinson's disease to Alzheimer's, cerebral palsy, epilepsy, and retardation. But more, they could be used to create models of what happens in the brain during addiction, depression, mania, and schizophrenia. And those with real imagination and hope, said Snyder, could envision a time when normal brain cells—and their chemistries—could be grown, modified, manipulated, and then implanted to restore or repair diseased or damaged brains.

With specialized colonies of laboratory-grown brain cells, surgeons might one day enhance, speed up, slow down, retard, or stop particular responses, memories, or feelings. In tandem with precision brain maps, genetic engineering, and delivery systems that cross the blood/brain barrier, normal brain cells might carry chemicals, drugs, and genes that regulate mood and behavior deep within the brain to repair holes; reprogram signals; and relieve depression, panic, schizophrenia, and a host of other mental illnesses.

Taking cell, gene, or drug implants, or remote-control stimulators, to the brain may represent the majority of "psychosurgery" of the future. Even now, advances in neuroscience are suggesting surgical techniques that could safely extend conventional psychiatric surgery to more of those who need it. For example, Nobel laureate David Baltimore, a molecular biologist and president of Rockefeller University, has developed transgenic mice, animals whose normal genome has been supplemented with genes that make vital brain chemicals such as serotonin. Serotonin plays a key role in obsessive-compulsive disorder and might one day be delivered "psychosurgically" to serotonin-depleted sites in the brains of OCD victims.

Neuroscientists now have the tools to exploit, as never before, means of watching both normal and abnormal brains in action. Functions we consider typical, like learning new verbs, and functions we consider mystical, like hallucinations and creativity. PET scans, especially, are revealing that very tiny clusters of brain cells are distinctly responsible for very particular actions and, therefore, accessible and amenable to precision repair and fine-tuning with chemical and surgical toolkits. Researchers are constructing all new models of behavior. Coupled with these new models is the notion that because the mind-brain combination governs behavior, the things people do—especially "wrong," "bad," or "inappropriate" things—should be as subject to definitive repair as any malfunctioning enterprise. Indeed, recent history has seen the medicalization of many behaviors once believed to be beyond the reach and interest of medical or surgical treatment, including alcoholism, promiscuity, aggression, pedophilia, homosexuality, drug abuse, and even shyness. And although the medical model tends to favor such nonpermanent means as drugs and talk therapies to treat these "ailments," the notion that treatment might be fast and definitive—i.e., surgical—is seductive.

No one can accurately gauge how fast new advances will come to the aid of patients, but the excitement and possibilities seen by the doctors and experimenters engaged in the work offer some insight into near-term possibilities—perhaps within the next decade. A catalog of some of the best conclude this chapter. But underpinning this enterprise are some fundamental ideas common to all of them and supported by a growing body of facts.

First, *all* disorders that affect the brain yield *neurologic, behavioral,* and *emotional* consequences. Neurologic are those we can think of as predominantly biological, chemical, anatomical, and mechanical. If you suffer brain damage in an auto accident, get viral encephalitis, take certain drugs, or inherit certain genes, brain tissue and cells are destroyed and along with them a part of the brain's ability to perform such tasks as receiving and sending signals to other parts of the brain and making and using important chemicals.

Behavioral consequences are actions others can observe and react to. A young man brain injured in any of the ways mentioned above may no longer do things he learned to do earlier in life, such as walk, talk, see, think in certain ways, get an erection, get out of the way of danger, or interact with others. Behaviorally, these changes may lead to other symptoms born of frustration, anger, depression, and mental and physical limitations.

Finally, there are emotional consequences of damage, disease, and disorder. Some, like severe forms of depression, can already be tracked to abnormal levels of certain chemicals in the brain, and miswired signal-carrying circuits, but the depression is—to the outside world and the patient—no different from the "blues," except they get worse and don't diminish. Other consequences include mania, rage, paranoia, severe jealously, obsessions, compulsiveness, anxiety, panic, and intense love and hate—exaggerations and intensifications of emotions we all share.

The second idea sustaining modern neuroscience is that the borders around all these consequences are not distinct, but blurred, intricately interwoven and interdependent, influencing each other to raise or lower particular responses and activities. At times of panic, for instance, our bodies discharge chemicals from the adrenal gland that in turn influence the activity of certain parts of the brain, leading to distortions of physical prowess, thinking and concentrating, sweating, and such emotions as fear. This "upstream-downstream" phenomenon is what is responsible for a 100-pound woman's sudden ability to lift a 3,200-pound car and free her child; or for our hearts to pound when we fall in love.

"Traditionally," writes Johns Hopkins's Snyder in his book, *Biological Aspects of Mental Disorders,* "there have been controversies between those espousing 'biological' and those favoring 'psychological' views of mental illness. In my perception, increased scientific understanding in both areas demonstrates convincingly that most of these disputes are built on mutual ignorance and misunderstanding." There is today, he argues, a "new biology of behavior."

The third idea supporting new concepts of psychosurgery and related surgical interventions is that by treating one symptom or consequence of a brain disorder, doctors may also be treating others, on purpose, or otherwise. As explained in Chapter Two, because our brains are organized in overlapping, intricately connected layers of cells and networks of cells, we have what an engineer might call an organ of redundant systems, with the *capability* of many functions widely spread around, or at least in touch. Emotions fall into this category, along with long-term memory, high-level learning, and problem solving.

"Several lines of knowledge are converging," says Guy McKhann, a Johns Hopkins neurologist who directs the Krieger Mind-Brain Institute. "We're finally getting out of what people in this business call 'boxology,' with experimental psychologists working in their 'box' of learning and thinking behavior, and biologists in their 'box' of physiology and genetics. Traditionally, the psychologist would set up his experiment to test how the mind works and the biologist would come along and say, 'Gee, that's an interesting phenomenon, so what part of the brain is involved?' and you'd get this blank look." Today, the tools are there to help the psychologist and the biologist talk to each other and swap information: PET scans light up areas of brain chemical activity, electronic implants reveal what parts of the brain do which thing, genetic recombination lets scientists manipulate and copy what the brain does, and computers unravel brain connections.

The brain, as we've said, works in systems, and each of those systems has several ways of telling scientists what they do and what goes wrong with them. Figuring out those systems means "getting into the clockworks." The idea isn't to watch the clockmaker make a broken clock run, but to watch clocks being made. One lover of metaphors saw the difference as a dishwashing problem. "A dishwasher can wash dishes much better than any human being ever could, and we made dishwashers by analyzing the different jobs that must be done—soaking, sudsing, rinsing, drying—and mimicking them. If they break, we can fix them, too. But dishwashers won't ever tell you a damn thing about how humans wash dishes. If we really want to improve human performance in washing dishes, *that's* the problem to solve."

The systems or "neural networks" brain scientists need to crack in order to get inside the clockworks are exquisitely complicated. One way of getting a fix on just how complicated is to picture a particular neuron in the visual system of the cerebral cortex and its "receptive" field, or areas from which it can receive electrical or chemical input from other neurons. This single neuron will respond to very specific stimuli. Call this the first-order neuron. Now picture a second neuron getting its input from, and depending on, collections of first-order neurons and think what and where the receptive fields for this second-order neuron might be. If you're recording these cells with chemical tracers or electrical pictures, you might be able, sometimes, to track, and after a while even predict, the step that goes from a first-order neuron to a second-order neuron. When you get to the third-order neuron, though, the cell is starting to have to take in and sort out more and more signals and more and more information.

In order to keep all the information being produced straight, working right, and packed into reasonable amounts of space, this third-order neuron has to integrate them, change them into complexes that are entirely different from anything it's taking in, and, in essence, make new information. It's like changing inventories of salt, sugar, flour, and shortening into stores of bread and cake. There's so much action among so many cells that the simple one-to-one relationship you started with is buried under layers of receptive fields. Now at least the tools are becoming available to gather and analyze "third-order" information involved in how our brains not only process visual images but also thoughts, feelings, and behavior. What's sure to follow is a map or blueprint of the clockworks themselves and the know-how to change or fix them if they are broken.

Over the past few years, psychologists, neurobiologists, and computer experts have also discovered a few of the strategies the brain uses to manage its vast neural networks and data banks. Potentially, the most useful are the parallel systems that operate the mind with an intricate dance of interpretation. PET scan studies by Marcus Raichle at Washington University in St. Louis, for instance, have shown that although there is a "language" center in the brain, the brain recruits separate sites to process words that are heard as against words that are seen or spoken. When "nonsense" words are flashed on a screen, moreover, the subject's brain processes these in yet another region.

Put another way, our brains have developed "shortcuts" to help us create order out of a chaotic world, and scientists are finding them. Bioengineer Leif Finkel of the University of Pennsylvania explains that in his view, our minds—unlike our brains—inhabit a "mixed realm" of reality and interpretation, which we can never consciously sort out. "Our cortex," he says poetically, "makes up stories about the world and softly hums them to us to keep us from getting scared at night." Poetry aside, computer "modelers" like Finkel are re-creating circuitry that, like neural networks, recognizes not just "reality" but context. One such network recognizes patterns of letters that form words with different shades of meaning in context.

Artificial intelligence—building robots or machines operated by "expert" software to perform certain tasks—is child's play compared with copying or understanding neural networks, but scientists are making headway in their efforts to find out how the brain "puts it all together." With the models that emerge from such studies, neurologists, psychiatrists, and neurosurgeons will be able to tell what information a neuron is sending out and to which other neurons up and down the line. They'll be able to predict where the action is and where it's going to wind up, permitting interventions to prevent or repair problems more precisely.

In sum, new technologies and new information will keep scientists running up the next scientific hill. Unquestionably, the experts interviewed told me, advances will create more opportunities for directly intervening in the workings of the minds and brains of patients with psychiatric illness or psychiatric symptoms linked to physical illness. Some of the advances are far from payoff; others already nearing headline status. All are at the cutting edge, the frontiers of neuroscience. Among them are the following.

GENE IMPLANTS AND GENE THERAPY

At the University of California at San Diego, Fred Gage is growing immortal cells that can be "transfected" with any gene in the hope of eventually transplanting them into the nervous system. The genes that make the business end of biochemicals, including neurotransmitters, are rapidly being sequenced and cloned; their precise amino acid makeup is being revealed. It's conceivable that implanting cells containing the genes that make chemicals that in turn block dopamine uptake in the brains of schizophrenics might in fact "cure" schizophrenia. Transfected cells might restore biochemical balance in the brains of people with bipolar disorder, or manic-depressive psychosis. Other cells might carry genes that can turn on or turn off, or turn up, or turn down other genes that are present, but not properly "tuned."

In related work, scientists at Yale University School of Medicine led by Neil Risch have begun studies that use genetic markers to detect sites on genes and chromosomes that contribute to certain psychiatric disorders. These are illnesses that seem to "run" in families—such as schizophrenia, obsessive-compulsive disease, manic-depressive psychosis, and panic disorder—leading scientists to suspect they have a strong genetic, or inherited, component. The International Human Genome Project designed to sequence and "map," or assign a site, on our chromosomes to all 50,000 to 100,000 genes is speeding their job. There already is evidence that an excess amount of genetic material on chromosome 5 is linked to schizophrenia and that the X, or female, chromosome carries some markers that point to genes for bipolar disease. Geneticists hope these markers—actually short strings of DNA, the basic building blocks of genes—will help them find people at risk for psychiatric illness early in their lives and eventually lead to treatments that replace, override, or disable faulty genes.

UNRAVELING THE NEUROLOGY AND CHEMISTRY OF BAD HABITS

Evidence mounts that a variety of what we usually call "bad habits," as well as classic obsessive-compulsive disorder, may involve the same abnormal brain circuitry. Specialists estimate that 2 to 3 percent of the U.S. population alone—that's up to 4 million Americans—have obsessive-compulsive disorder and *related* disorders, including bowel and urinary tract obsessions, eating disorders, compulsive gambling, compulsive sexual behavior, and hypochondriasis.

A recent piece of evidence for a common biochemical link, published in the *New England Journal of Medicine* in August 1989, is that a drug that helps people who obsessively pull their hair also works with other forms of OCD, and the scientists are planning to experiment with the drug on chronic nail biters, face pickers, and smokers. The drugs are known as serotonergic, or responsive to or stimulated by the neurotransmitter serotonin, and they include the drug clomipramine, which is effective against many cases of OCD. That chemical profile suggests that portions of the brain rich in serotonin receptors may be involved in illnesses long considered to be exclusively psychiatric rather than physical. In addition, PET scans suggest abnormalities in the frontal lobes, caudate nucleus, and basal ganglia of patients with OCD; and MRI shows differences in frontal lobe white matter in OCD and Tourette's disease patients.

Michael Jenike and his coworkers Robert L. Martuza and Tom Ballantine at Massachusetts General Hospital performed PET scans of patients with obsessive-compulsive disease to see if they could find differences in the brains of those patients. The scans, which show how areas of the brain use energy-supplying sugar, revealed abnormalities of sugar metabolism in the caudate nuclei and the frontal lobes of OCD patients. MRI and CT scans, which reveal anatomy rather than biochemistry, have further suggested that in obsessive-compulsive disorder there is a circuit that runs in and out of the thalamus, frontal lobes, and cortex that also is involved, regulated by several neurotransmitters: dopamine, GABA, serotonin, and glutamate.

Old-style lobotomies and today's more limited limbic system operations help OCD patients by removing some of the regulatory connections, but these modern studies support the idea that drugs and even more precise surgical lesions at the affected brain sites may offer some patients who cannot be helped any other way a permanent control or cure. Says psychiatrist Jenike, "understanding the pathophysiology of these disorders will benefit our patients and may also shed light on the biology of certainty, doubt, motivation, and satisfaction."

GROWING NEW TISSUE IN THE BRAIN

Over the last ten years, research suggests that neurons and other cells in the central nervous system can regenerate if the environment is right. Scientists have in fact discovered chemical factors, such as nerve growth factor, that stimulate proteins to sprout. Snyder used some of these substances to help his brain cell line get started. In animal experiments, fetal brain tissue has been transplanted to adult animals and grown there. Dr. Albert Aguayo of Canada's McGill University has used pieces of rat nerve to rebuild connections between spinal cords and brains in adult rats who have a condition similar to paraplegia or quadriplegia. That has led to hope that severed spinal cord cells and brain damage can someday be repaired by first growing, then implanting, viable brain tissue. Or by implanting long-acting capsules of the chemical factors that stimulate existing cells to divide and multiply.

Jerry Silver, a neuroanatomist at Case Western Reserve University, and Ionannis Yannas of the Massachusetts Institute of Technology have surgically implanted a silicon tube containing a biodegradable gel to create a "bridge" on which nerve tissue has grown across severed rat nerves. Similar approaches for transplants and regeneration may someday be possible for quadriplegics and victims of Alzheimer's and Parkinson's diseases. They might also be used to repair "holes" in the brain made by injury or by surgeons removing abnormal tissue and circuitry.

Fetal nerve tissue already has been implanted in at least two men with severe cases of Parkinson's disease, one in Sweden and one in the United States. Reports say both can now walk without canes and their hands have stopped shaking. Apparently the fetal cells can do what the patients' nerve cells have lost the ability to do: secrete the neurotransmitter dopamine. Fetal cell transplants—if they prove effective and safe—offer a tempting way to get a variety of neurotransmitters and other drugs into target sites in the limbic brain, another path for psychosurgery in the future.

UNDERSTANDING THE EMOTIONAL AND BEHAVIORAL CONSEQUENCES OF STROKE

Antonio Culebras, professor of neurology at the State University of New York in Syracuse, has studied six patients with a bizarre sleep disorder marked by pinching, kicking, screaming, or leaping from bed so violently they sometimes injure themselves and others. They also have nightmares and confrontational dreams. MRI scans of these patients' brains revealed lesions caused by small strokes. Culebras suspected strokes because for decades, scientists have been able to induce a condition similar to his patients' in laboratory animals by deliberately causing lesions in a specific area of the brain stem. Says Culebras: "Our study suggests that injury from stroke to the equivalent area of the human brain has similar results."

Research conducted by Robert Robinson, M.D., while at Johns Hopkins, has forged other connections between emotions and stroke and by doing so may help guide surgery and drug therapy safely around or through these connections in the future. The results of Robinson's studies revealed that the incidence of depression is much higher than expected in some stroke patients, particularly left brain stroke victims, suggesting that stroke is one of nature's "backward psychosurgeries," and that the damage, or lesions, made in the cortex by a stroke is coordinated with parts of the limbic system. Robinson and his coworkers also found that left brain stroke victims can feel depressed for years after a stroke, making them uncooperative in rehabilitation programs and creating a history of being difficult and nasty. Not surprisingly, antidepressive medication has helped many of his patients enormously, despite resistance from conventional psychiatrists who keep insisting that poststroke depression is transient—based on the simple fact of having had a stroke—and should not be medically treated because the drugs may "cover up" or delay boot-strap operations for self-recovery and coping with reality.

But beyond the clinical applications of his work, these studies also support the hypothesis that the brain's two sides have evolved with special circuits and tissues for different emotional experiences. By examining the brain with CT scans after a stroke and relating anatomy to results on a series of psychiatric, mood, and neurological tests, scientists learned that the worst stroke-related depressions occurred when the lesions were in the front part of the left brain. "The closer to the frontal areas, the more likely was the emotional effect," said Robinson. In contrast, patients who had damage in the front part of the right half of the brain were those who showed inappropriate gaiety and almost complete apathy toward the seriousness of their disability.

MAPPING THE BRAIN AND EMOTIONS

The first efforts to map the anatomy of an emotion probably took place in the Middle Ages when doctors taught that "humors" or body fluids were the cause of mood. Too much "bile" and the patient was depressed; too much "blood" translated into optimism and cheer. But the first modern-day stab at it came in 1968 at

Washington University in St. Louis when scientists put an infusion of the chemical sodium lactate into a normal volunteer undergoing a PET scan and triggered a full-blown panic attack. They were able to link the attack to abnormal patterns of blood flow, blood volume, and use of oxygen in the brain's temporal lobe. When that work was published in 1984 in *Nature,* it caused a revolution in the thinking about mental illness. Here was solid evidence that at least one mental illness laid down specific neurological tracks.

Today, using advanced PET scans to watch the brain conduct its chemical chores, scientists are unlocking the similarities and differences between the normal everyday anxiety anyone might feel en route to giving a speech and panic disorder, the terror that strikes without warning, without control, and without an outside event to trigger it. (As one patient at Washington University described his attacks, "It was like having a heart attack. I could hardly breathe." He withdrew from all social life and normal activities out of a developing fear he'd have more attacks.) Drs. Marcus Raichle and Peter Fox have discovered that unlike people who get normal anxiety, the estimated 1 million Americans with panic disorder have more blood flow and metabolic activity in the right side of the brain than the left, even when they are calm, but that both normal and abnormal anxiety share a common path involving the cortex, or thinking brain.

In one series of experiments, they studied people who are virtually disabled by anxiety attacks, people who are clearly at special risk, or vulnerable, with relatively minor triggers. It's enough to just tell these individuals they are participating in a study that requires them to get a very painful electric shock to the thumb. The shock is not given at that point; they simply let the person anticipate the pain. Most people would get anxious from this, but this subset of people get totally disabled from it. The scientists then asked, what happens in what part of the brain to these people that does not happen in others? The answer: PET scans showed heavy blood flow in the left temporal lobe especially. What they discovered was a narrow strip of brain tissue involved in a mood—anxiety.

The same kind of anxiety could also be triggered in this sub-group with infusions of lactate, a chemical salt that apparently either enhances the sensitivity of some brain cells or turns off antianxiety chemicals. Fox and other scientists have shown that, in animals at least, they can chemically block the panic attacks by adding known chemicals that block lactate uptake by certain brain cells. Not surprisingly, tranquilizers already known to help patients with panic disorder turn out to be related to chemicals that block the uptake of lactate. "In the long run," says Raichle, "if we define the predisposing neuroanatomy of the disease, we can begin to ... understand what kinds of drugs would be effective ... because ... neurons talk to other neurons through receptors and transmitters." And so, too, perhaps devise surgical interventions, not only for panic but also for phobias, addictions, and other disorders of thinking and behaving.

Since the St. Louis studies were first reported, PET, MRI, CT, and other computer-generated imaging machines have given scientists unprecedented pictures of how anatomy (structure) and behavior (function) link up in the mind and brain. Studies on monkeys, for example, show 32 areas of the cerebral cortex and 305 separate circuits involved with vision alone. All these circuits were precisely pinpointed with PET scans that watch how blood flows through the brain and how the brain uses sugar and other nutrients. They do this by measuring gamma rays emitted by radioactive tracers attached to substances such as blood or glucose as they move through the brain. The studies also used MRI, which lights up specific brain regions as human subjects move, speak, recognize words and colors, or do other tasks.

Closing in on harder scientific evidence that the geography and chemistry of the brain and its cells are the keys to much mental and emotional illness in humans, the scientists see the time coming when each person with an unwanted behavior will have his or her own behavioral brain map to guide treatment—drug, surgical, or a combination of the two. Among the possible applications of such knowledge: surgical introduction of long-term infusions of drugs into the brain, electrode implants that can be self-activated to ward off the attack, and surgically created lesions that permanently damage the receptors. "Our findings," report Raichle and his coworkers in the June 1989 issue of *Archives of General Psychiatry*, "may also be relevant to [the] ... fear commonly experienced in association with temporal lobe seizures and ... anxiety attacks in association with [brain] pathology." These same regions may also be in play in people with unusual displays of uncertainty, helplessness, shyness, or paranoia.

Fox and Raichle have also looked at brain response to anxiety-provoking situations such as pain and have mapped increases in blood flow in the temporal lobes that result from those situations. And they have used PET scans to watch how the brain processes individual words, demonstrating that the brain operates differently when the word is read from when it is heard. The implications for training the deaf and helping the reading impaired are profound. But even more profound is what such studies are teaching neuroscientists about the complex learning, memory, and psychological links in the thinking brain, or cortex. And given the links already known between what our brains can do and how we perceive our world, it may be that they will shed intense new light on why some people have a distorted view of the world, why they think differently, and why we may need to view such disorders as schizophrenia, multiple personalities, and antisocial behavior in very original ways.

One of the most fascinating series of related studies in this field comes from Michael Gazzaniga, a psychiatrist and neuroscientist at Dartmouth Medical School, famous for his so-called split-brain research. Taking advantage of patients whose corpus callosum has been severed by accident, birth defect, or surgery (to treat epilepsy and brain tumors), he has shown that the brain contains "modules" that separate functions with a high degree of precision, yet that communicate with each other at certain levels.

The first experiments on such patients suggested that each half of the brain operates independently and can't communicate with the other half. For instance, in split-brain patients, if you electrically stimulate a joint on one finger in a way that the patient can't see it and the patient is asked to indicate where the stimulation was with the thumb of the same hand, they can do so as long as the stimulus and response are on the same hand. But if you stimulate the joint on one finger and ask the patient to find the corresponding point of stimulation on the other hand, the split-brain patient can't do it except by chance. Keep in mind that the left brain is considered to be the verbal, analytical, and dominant side, responsible for language, speech, writing, mathematical ability, and control of the right side of the body, so that you write with your right hand in most cases. The right brain is considered the artistic side, able to discriminate shapes and colors and vision. The right brain interprets the world in terms of what we call imagination; it's the receiver and identifier of spaces, shapes, and places and of a sense of where we are and where we've been, the nonverbal colorful part of the brain. A patient who has only a left hemisphere can speak and write with his right hand and feel and sense things, but he cannot reproduce shapes or understand music. If this patient had a ball hidden from his view but held in his right hand, he could say what it was but if it was held in his left hand he could not say what it was but could detect it amid square blocks and shoestrings. He could recognize the ball in his left hand but couldn't talk about it.

Gazzaniga's new studies, however, suggest that the two hemispheres of the brain forge communications links and swap information, especially when complex learning and memory activities are involved. One implication is that the neural memory of skills, behavior, and perhaps emotions might be transferable from one part of the brain to another. In one test, a patient before split-brain surgery was asked to handle an irregularly shaped wire figure he could not see and then asked to select it from a group of four other wire figures. The patient could do this with either hand, suggesting that this information is distributed to the right hemisphere from information arrived at in her left brain from the right hand and from the right brain for the left hand. After the back half of her callosum was cut, she could not name objects placed in the left hand because fibers her brain needed to transfer touch and feel information were severed and so the left hand/right brain system literally did not know what the right hand/left brain knew. And the patient could no longer do the wire figure task with either hand. Because this patient could do the task before surgery, in the normally intact system, the right brain must have the ability to solve this kind of problem when connected to the left brain. This in turn suggests that the left brain normally helps the right brain do certain "right brain" tasks and vice versa.

How this kind of information illuminates mental illness and the emotional pathways in the limbic system is just beginning to be realized. But there already is evidence that the disordered thinking, delusions, and fears exhibited by many of the mentally ill will turn out to have their roots in these "communications" problems. In neuroscience studies, says Gazzaniga, there is a "tendency ... to overlook possible mechanisms related to the truly psychological dimension of human life." Gazzaniga looks straight at them. One means he developed is called a simultaneous concept test, in which a patient is shown two pictures, one just to the left hemisphere (through the right eye) and one just to the right, and asked to choose from among an array of pictures placed in full view those associated with the pictures he only saw with the left brain (right eye) or right brain (left eye).

A picture of a chicken claw, for instance, was flashed to the left brain and a snow scene to the right. In the full-view array of pictures, there were a chicken and a shovel. The "correct" association is to link the chicken with the chicken claw and shovel for the snow scene. But the split-brain subject chose the shovel with the left hand and the chicken with the right. When asked why, his left brain replied, out loud, "Oh that's simple. The chicken claw goes with the chicken and you need a shovel to clean out the chicken shed." In this case, the left brain "saw" the response of the left hand and interpreted that response into a *context* that fit in with its area of expertise—an area that did not include any information about the snow scene flashed to the left brain.

Gazzaniga translates these observations into insights about behavior and mood. Mood shifts, he once wrote, can be triggered by manipulating the disconnected right brain. A positive mood shift triggered by the right brain causes the left brain to "explain" its experience in a positive way and or a negative mood shift in a negative way. Perhaps a variety of psychological disturbances that are initially produced by endogenous errors in cerebral metabolism, such as those known to be associated with panic attacks, also produce a different "feeling" that must be interpreted by the brain. And "each individual's interpretation, unique to their own past and present psychological history, is then stored in memory and becomes powerfully determinant in the content of an individual's ongoing consciousness." Even if the internal events are healed through drugs or time, the brain remembers its altered mood. In extreme cases, such as a panic attack, phobias sometimes develop. The phobia may be the brain's explanation and interpretation of the altered biological state and can stick around long after the panic attack is successfully treated with sedatives.

TRANSIENT PSYCHOSURGERY

Pain, stress, and anxiety all have similar nerve pathways and biochemical components despite the fact that most people view stress and anxiety to be "psychosocial" in origin and pain strictly biological. All three responses are regulated by areas of the brain associated with a part of the limbic system that produces about 70 percent of the brain's supply of norepinephrine, a neurotransmitter linked to irritability, alertness, and anxiety. Excess norepinephrine can trigger panic, high blood pressure, sweat, and nausea. Its effects can be dampened by endorphins made in the pituitary gland. Endorphins are the body's natural opiates, produced when there is too much norepinephrine. In chronic stress, the body may burn out its ability to recognize and attend to repeated "hits," often generating endorphins that put the mind out of its misery. Compulsive eating and gambling may emerge from damage to our ability to respond to too high levels of norepinephrine produced at times of stress.

In TENS, researchers have found that mild current produces a jolt of ß-endorphins in the cerebrospinal fluid that affects the emotional centers of the brain more than the pain centers and alleviates depression and anxiety as well as pain. As a form of "transient" or "temporary" psychosurgery, TENS may have value in phobias; panic attacks; addictions, including gambling; and any medical conditions in which symptoms are exacerbated by stress and anxiety, including irritable bowel syndrome, diabetes, and high blood pressure. By intervening in a part of the circuit that is easy to reach, TENS is able to modify more complex systems.

DIRECT-TO-BRAIN THERAPY FOR DRUG ADDICTION AND VIOLENCE

Because of the political, legal, and moral controversies involved in any effort to treat behaviors that society considers criminal, research in this area poses ethical as well as medical problems. Nevertheless there is evidence that for some people who abuse addictive drugs and commit violent acts, surgical and medical treatment might benefit them and the communities in which they live.

Scientists don't have a clear idea of what happens in the brain in somebody who's addicted to, say, cocaine, or what the real changes are that send the addict on the road to self-destruction. One hypothesis, however, is that taking coke "cranks up" the production of dopamine and the whole dopamine system in some parts of the brain and may even increase the number of activated dopamine receptors. Or it may be that in some individuals, the dopamine system already is wound up. Then the only way to meet the demand for dopamine is to get it from outside sources. It's possible, say those who advance the dopaminergic theory of cocaine addiction, to treat the addict with a safer, less objection-able form of dopamine, as with the L-Dopa or other drugs given to Parkinson's disease patients. An alternative few talk about is surgery to damage dopamine receptors, which might not only modify the unwanted behavior (taking drugs, getting high, stealing to support the habit) but also "cure" the biological need for the drug.

The same kinds of studies under way with anxiety and panic disorders are also on the planning board for aggression, the nervous system's expression of fear and response to threats that in humans often comes out as violence against others. Studies on animals and in patients with damage to the temporal lobes clearly demonstrate that there are parts of the brain directly involved in the control—or lack of control—of violence. Surgery on the amygdala and cingulum, as we saw in Chapter Four, can stop violent outbursts by damping down the aggressive controls in the brain.

Studies of certain epilepsy patients *between* seizures suggest that temporal lobe epilepsy leaves its victims with much greater sensitivity to many emotions, moral issues, intense anger, and slights or violations of principle. Religious fanaticism is more frequent in these patients than in the general population. When such people do commit violent acts, they may do so with a clear conscience but express sincere sorrow at their behavior afterward. According to David Bear, director of neuropsychiatry at the Vanderbilt University School of Medicine, damage to one part of the frontal lobe—the dorsal portion—results in apathy and lack of motivation to act on one's own. Damage to the undersurface results in reflex emotional response, periods of irritability, and violent response to even minor provocations. Victims may know the rules but simply don't consider them. They're impulsive and casual about the consequences, exhibiting a "so what" attitude. In many aggressive individuals, Bear says, there may be no obvious epilepsy or lesions, but subtle impairment of the hypothalamus, amygdala, or frontal cortex.

These emotional brain areas do not reveal their subtle damage to ordinary neurologic examinations, Bear notes. That would require studies with PET, MRI, and CT scans that can "see" at a microscopic and molecular level. But he points out that the mass murderer Henry Lee Lukas has documented lesions of the frontal and temporal lobes. There is also evidence that the James Hinckley, the would-be assassin of former President Ronald Reagan, likewise had abnormal temporal lobes. "It is certainly not my suggestion that all human aggression has a primary organic or structural basis," Bear wrote in a Harvard Medical School magazine in 1989. But that is part of it, he said.

As the next chapter reveals, the psychosurgical treatment of violence and other antisocial behavior is one possible outcome of the research frontiers, an outcome with more potential for abuse than most critics will tolerate.

CHAPTER SEVEN

THE LAW-AND-ORDER LOBBY

*There is a new [sic] medical procedure which is humane, safe
and permanent, one which will eliminate the violent criminals from our society, reduce our prison population by 10 to
15 percent and provide for early release of all individuals....
This procedure is frontal lobotomy.*

—FORMER REPUBLICAN STATE REPRESENTATIVE
DALE ERICKSON (COLO.), JUNE 1989

Is he serious? Is he for real?

—REPUBLICAN STATE REPRESENTATIVE
CAROL TAYLOR-LITTLE (COLO.), JUNE 1989

Dale Erickson is serious and he is for real.

By the late 1960s, psychosurgery as an instrument of social control seemed to most people a dead issue. But not to all.
"Lobotomized criminals," Erickson says, "would not have to be
cared for by the taxpayers and instead of more prisons, the
patients could be released to work for taxpayers and government
and private businesses." He openly favors this "slave labor" to deal
with the twin evils of lawlessness and prison costs, arguing that
prisoners are by definition "slaves," because they have no—or at
least fewer—constitutional rights. There's nothing in the federal
or Colorado state constitution that prohibits the use of lobotomy,
he argues, and lobotomy is a serious means of dealing with hard-

ened criminals in a less cruel, more humane way than incarceration for life or the death penalty. Erickson admits that most lobotomy patients could not function without close supervision. "But they would require nurses, not armed guards. They could be servants, like children, who can wash cars, do farm work, and so on. They should be punished, not coddled, and hard work is the best punishment."

In legislation submitted to the Colorado legislature, he proposes an "Adopt-a-Con" program in which social service agencies and prisons would place convicts with families to do chores. "It's better than 40 years with no parole in a bad-ass prison. Their return to society would be humane and would serve as a *great* deterrent. Any kid would see a lobotomized slave and say 'Not me, I'll never break the law.'" In a letter drafted to the governor and every state legislator of Colorado, Erickson argues that you "cannot legislate morality," so the solution to overcrowded prisons and violent crime rests in more imaginative solutions like his.

It is tempting to simply dismiss Erickson as a fool and his brand of "law and order by knife" as the fantasies of an aging paranoiac with too much money and too little regard for civil rights. Few accept his false claim that lobotomies are today "accepted as standard medical practice for the violently insane in our sanitariums ... so why not violent and dangerous criminals?" Yet, surprisingly—perhaps, alarmingly—few have aggressively faced him down.

The one-term Colorado state representative (1984 to 1986) and descendent of Scandinavian immigrants grew up in the Minnesota north woods, attended a one-room school in the 1930s, and nurtures a John Birch Society brand of conservative politics. In many ways, he embodies the American values and character lionized in the Reagan years: rugged individualism, can-do pragmatism, discipline, and anger at those who don't pull their weight. The son of a commercial fisherman, he owns a prospering glass company and a cattle and sheep ranch; has a lot of money and considerable goodwill from years of community service as a scoutmaster, Little League coach, and former president of the Chamber of Commerce in Ft. Lupton; and he is a good old boy in local Republican circles.

Erickson's extremist proposal spices the ongoing debate over psychosurgery's value with justifiable fear and loathing. It telegraphs the potent peril psychosurgery still carries and jeopardizes the renewed interest in the legitimate surgical treatment of mental illness. Frighteningly, some version of his views on dealing with violent criminals, social misfits, and other burdens win grudging support from less radical and more thoughtful quarters, partly because the criminal justice system isn't very good at predicting dangerous behavior in parolees and partly because psychiatrists frequently publicize the heavy role of mental illness in antisocial behavior. "Psychiatrists already are used as agents of the state to incarcerate and punish as well as treat," says forensic psychiatrist Jeffrey Janofsky. "The perception of the law-and-order lobby is that we are nuts, and that society is out of control and someone needs to take control." In the preface to his 1977 book, *Psychosurgery and the Medical Control of Violence,* forensic psychiatrist and lawyer Samuel I. Shuman notes that "throughout history, 'medicine' has been an instrument of social policy and physicians have been involved in the control and suppression of social deviance." The medical profession, for instance, has granted or refused access to safe abortions with an eye to political consequences; it insisted for decades that women who worked outside the home put their health at risk. It conducts executions by lethal injection, supports involuntary commitments, and has promoted sterilizations among the poor.

To one degree or another, members of the law-and-order lobby, including state legislators, lawyers, psychiatrists, surgeons, and criminologists, are frustrated with rising crime rates and the costs of prisons and hospitals for the criminally insane. The failure of criminal rehabilitation efforts is trumpeted often in the press, and privately many admit that such an environment offers fertile ground for extremist initiatives. "Lots of careful, respectable people have done real stupid things," says Robert A. Burt, J.D., professor of law at Yale University and for decades a critic of medical "solutions" to social problems bought at the expense of civil rights.

While people may decisively reject Erickson's proposal, they do not necessarily reject the use of lobotomy's safer, less mutilating approximations, amygdalotomy and cingulotomy, if in fact they could calm the brain's centers of violence in selected patients. Giving aid and comfort to this idea are relatively ambiguous laws and regulations. Although "experimental" surgery and other treatments are generally prohibited among prisoners and inmates of hospitals for the criminally insane, court cases are still brought to challenge outright bans. If psychosurgery is ever deemed standard rather than experimental, the picture will become more cloudy.

Burt and Shuman, a professor of law at Wayne State University when he wrote *Control of Violence*, were both key figures in the one case directly dealing with psychosurgery as an abusive tool of social control ever brought to trial in the United States. In the end, the court did not completely reject the idea of behavior control with surgery, and Burt and Shuman both believe the decision reflects persistent ambivalence in the courts about the rights of individuals versus the rights of society to be safe.

The details of the case, known as *Kaimowitz v. Dept. of Mental Health*, or the Detroit psychosurgery trial, are worth reviewing. Shuman was counsel to the physicians in the trial that pitted a lawyer named Gabe Kaimowitz against the Michigan Department of Mental Health, which wanted to proceed with limited psychosurgery experiments on certain prisoners.

The case began in 1972 when a neurosurgeon affiliated with Wayne State University Medical School, Ernst Rodin, and his colleague Jacques Gottlieb of the Lafayette Clinic, a facility of the Michigan Department of Mental Health, filed a proposal for the study of treatment of uncontrollable aggression to be funded by the legislature for that fiscal year. In their proposal, they outlined a comparative study of amygdalotomy and male hormone suppressants in patients committed to institutions for the criminally insane because of uncontrollable violence. To get into the study, patients had to be male, to be aged 25 or older; to have been inmates for 5 or more years sentenced for aggressive behavior; to be resistant to all other treatment; to possess an IQ over 80; to have a sense of remorse and desire to stop their violent behavior; and lastly, to be able to give informed consent and get consent from relatives or guardians.

One of the state hospitals in which Rodin and Gottlieb sought candidates was Ionia State, which housed a group of about 25 patients all considered criminal sexual psychopaths. One of the 25, a man named Louis Smith (referred to in the court record as John Doe), had been committed there in January 1955, without trial after being charged with the murder and rape of a student nurse at the state hospital where he had been confined as a mental patient for 17 years. Burt, who represented John Doe when the case eventually came to trial, recalled in a recent interview what happened next:

> According to accounts, Doe was the only inmate who volunteered to enter the study and Rodin, or rather his staff, made clear to him that if he was accepted in the experiment, having the operation would not mean automatic release. No promises were made about that and they were very explicit. They said that if the operation were a success and he were cured, however, the cure would be taken into account. The inmate was taken to Lafayette Clinic in Detroit, where Wayne State University School of Medicine was located, and prepared for the surgery. He'd already had depth electrodes put in his brain to locate the tissue believed to be the site of his rages, when a local lawyer who had been very much involved in mental health reform issues found out about it. He created a blaze of media publicity and brought suit to stop the experiment from going forward.

The local lawyer was a man named Gabe Kaimowitz, and he brought a writ of *habeas corpus*. He had never met John Doe, but, as Burt recalled, "his premise was, to put it kind of crudely, that anybody who would agree to have his brain scrambled must be crazy, and if you're crazy, you're not competent to consent. A catch-22." Moreover, Burt said, Kaimowitz believed that the whole consent effort with Doe was coercive, "since the man already was a virtual prisoner." Kaimowitz would also base his case on the fact that as a taxpayer in the state of Michigan, his tax dollars were being illegally spent to perform this experiment because it was in and on behalf of a state institution.

In the publicity that followed, the state pulled the plug on the entire research project, but the decision to proceed to trial was made because Rodin and Gottlieb insisted they had a right to do such procedures and they wanted to affirm the scientific validity of their proposal. At that point, the court decided Doe needed a personal lawyer, because Kaimowitz had not met him and had brought the suit without asking the subject. Burt, who was then professor of law at the University of Michigan, was appointed, along with Francis A. Allen, the dean of the Michigan law school. Shuman was called in to represent Rodin and Gottlieb.

In his first meeting with Doe, Burt tried to determine what Doe really wanted:

> I met him, talked with him, and he told me he felt there was some-
> thing wrong with his brain function. He recalled that eighteen years
> earlier, he had murdered a nurse in Ionia and after doing that had sex-
> ual intercourse with her body. A really horrible crime, but he was
> never actually convicted of it because until 1968 a law in Michigan
> allowed such individuals to be classified as criminal sexual psychopaths
> and in effect imprisoned forever or until cured. In any event, my con-
> clusion was that this was not a terrific fellow. He also told me about the
> subjective surges of violence and he found the idea of the blame being
> in his damaged brain appealing and the reason he volunteered for the
> surgery. He was in fact a very smart fellow. He said he knew no
> promises were being made, but he also knew that if he were coopera-
> tive and if indeed this operation cured the violent urges, it could help
> him get out. He was very clear on all of this and wanted to go forward.
>
> I said to him, "Look if it turned out that your original commitment
> under the criminal sexual psychopath act was illegal, would you want
> me to pursue that, to get you released without the operation?" and it
> took him about one second to say, "Sure, if you can do that." Well, in
> fact, I did get him released on that ground in March 1973. I found that
> the old 1968 statute was unconstitutional and the court agreed and he
> was released.

Wisely, the Michigan Department of Mental Health declined to seek civil commitment of Doe; they could not prove that he was dangerous to himself or others, because except for the one killing 18 years earlier, he had been involved in no other violence than what Burt termed "garden-variety" quarrels.

But Michigan felt the general issue was significant: The use of inmates in prisons or mental hospitals as potential subjects was critical in a whole variety of experiments. Thus, although the issue of John Doe was moot, the Department of Mental Health asked the court to go forward with the case and judge whether it is possible for anyone involuntarily confined in a state institution—prison or mental—to give adequate informed consent to participate in psychosurgery. Said Burt:

> If the answer were yes, then it would be legal in Michigan to undertake experiments on the brain of an adult if ... the procedure is designed to relieve behavior that is either personally tormenting to the patient or so profoundly disruptive that the patient cannot live safely in society. The trial was lengthy and there were all kinds of witnesses—neurosurgeons on both sides of the debate—on the scientific merits of the procedure and experts in bioethical matters arguing about consent. Among them were Dr. Bertram Brown, head of the National Institute of Mental Health, and Dr. Peter Breggin, a Washington, D.C., psychiatrist who has made a career of fanatical opposition to psychosurgery.
>
> The testimony suggested that the surgery in question was experimental, that little was known about it, and that there was growing concern about violence, so much so that a national commission was appointed by the late-President Lyndon Johnson under the chairmanship of Johns Hopkins University president Milton Eisenhower with fifty consultants in law, sociology, criminology, government, social psychiatry, and psychology.

Doe testified as well, about the process he had been through in regard to giving consent. The court ruled that Doe could not possibly have given adequate informed consent and outlawed the experiment on that basis in all Michigan state institutions. The opinion was very influential, effectively banning psychosurgery in state institutions throughout the country.

Unfortunately, legal experts say, *Kaimowitz* did not settle the issue nor did it kill the possibility of psychosurgery for violent criminals. While the jury may have come in for John Doe, it is still very much out with respect to surgical treatment of socially undesirable behavior. The *Kaimowitz* decision only protects those who are involuntarily confined. If you're not and you're just a member of the general public, the protection you have is whatever the institutional review board in the institution involved says it is. But perhaps more troubling for those who fear the abuse of psychosurgery is the fact that operations *are* used to stop aggression in selected inmate-patients. The stated goal is to better the quality of life for inmates and perhaps gain their freedom; but the line between "treatment" and "punishment," between help for the patient and ease for the prison system, is blurry.

Beyond ambiguous court decisions, what also keeps the surgery-for-violence idea from total oblivion are the writings and studies of neurosurgeons Vernon Mark and William Sweet of Harvard medical school and Boston psychiatrist Frank Ervin.

In 1967, just after the Detroit race riots that summer, the three wrote a letter to the *Journal of the American Medical Association* suggesting that urban rioting required extensive studies of individuals who participated, and perhaps psychosurgical treatment for those with "low violence thresholds." They offered reviews of case histories that suggested that people who commit arson, assault, and sniping have a high rate of brain wave abnormalities and that there was something "peculiar about the violent slum dweller that differentiates him from his peaceful neighbor"—focal lesions in the brain.

In a 1970 book, *Violence and the Brain,* and in subsequent articles published in 1973 and 1974, they presented evidence that psychosurgery—specifically lesions made in the amygdala and other parts of the limbic system—could become an important tool to reduce and control violence in the United States, declaring that much if not most of the violence in U.S. society was caused by a "dyscontrol" syndrome, a brain pathology caused by electrical firestorms in the temporal lobes of victims. Although such people do not necessarily have seizures, their abnormalities could be revealed with modern electroencephalograms and other technology. Moreover, they recommended tests on nonviolent, nondiseased limbic brains to diagnose who might have a "tendency" to "impulsive violence."

Their views resonated for a public frightened by and fed up with violence and antisocial behavior on a massive scale, exacerbated by poverty, drugs, and homelessness, as well as the perceived failure of psychotherapy and prison rehabilitation programs for chronic offenders. Dismissing critics who raised the specter of tyrannical government control of submissive populations, they countered that if indeed medical science could produce a technology capable of that scenario, it would in all likelihood have devices to block its use for such purposes as well. They frequently pointed out that tranquilizers and other drugs already posed a bigger threat of mind control. "The great hope of emotional brain research," they wrote, "is that it will free us from our present tyrannies."

The scientific evidence supporting some of Mark's and Ervin's claims was thin at best—there is no evidence that "much" or "most" violence, for example, springs from brain pathology or that limited psychosurgery can safely cure it. But even their critics acknowledged that there were some data to support their view. And some of the law-and-order community ran with the idea that medical science can defeat crime and violence well into the 1960s, 1970s, and 1980s. Consider:

- In February 1968, some of the events later publicized in Ken Kesey's 1973 novel *One Flew Over the Cuckoo's Nest* occurred in a maximum psychiatric prison intended for diagnosis, treatment, and research on prisoner volunteers at Vacaville prison. Three inmates with violent seizures underwent brain surgery for "behavioral" control. A less immediate agenda was to see if the surgery could rehabilitate them.

As M. Hunter Brown, a California neurosurgeon who supported psychosurgery, told the *National Enquirer* in 1972, "[a] person convicted of a violent crime should have the chance for a corrective operation.... Each violent young criminal incarcerated from 20 years to life costs taxpayers perhaps $100,000. For roughly $6,000, society can provide medical treatment which will transform him into a responsible, well-adjusted citizen."

• Michigan proposed its Lafayette Clinic experiments and the California Department of Corrections planned a program to locate brain tissue that could be the "site" of violent behavior and to operate on that site if they found it. It sought $300,000 from the U.S. Department of Justice's Law Enforcement Assistance Administration and $189,000 from the state of California.

• Medical journals published articles from world-class scientists suggesting that violent tendencies might be inherited via an extra Y chromosome in some males, and the National Institute of Mental Health gave Mark, Ervin, and Sweet a $500,000 grant to continue their work.

• In 1972 in California, then-Governor Ronald Reagan set up the Center for the Study and Reduction of Violence. Headed by Louis Jolyn West, it planned epidemiological studies of child abuse, homicide, and suicide in the young and sought ways of predicting pathological outbursts of violence; it looked for cultural clues to sex offenses and drug- and alcohol-related violence and examined animal models of violence.

• In February 1989, 150 leading scientists and engineers met for the Second International Conference on Peace Through Mind-Brain Science at Hamamatsu City in Japan.

Their mission, according to a news release issued on the subject, is "to promote the scientific study of brain mechanisms involved in destructive and violent behavior, as well as those related to loving and creative behavior." The release goes on to note that the specific objectives of the sponsoring organizations in Japan were (1) to develop the concept that peace will depend on a better scientific understanding of the human brain and its role in behavior; (2) to facilitate scientific and technological advances in the peaceful application of photonics—the science and technology of light (optics, lasers, and computer imaging machines) to the solution of human problems by providing new ways of looking at the human brain as we think, feel, and act; and (3) to facilitate international communication among basic and clinical neuroscientists, makers and users of photonics technology, scientists, and the public; and scientists, political leaders, and policymakers. Among the institutions represented were Merck, Siemens, General Electric, Suntory, Japanese electronics firms, Johns Hopkins University, Washington University in St. Louis, University of London, University of Pennsylvania, and University of California at Berkeley, as well as education and research institutes in the Soviet Union, Sweden, Canada, Switzerland, and Japan.

• In a complicated Supreme Court decision in February 1990 (*Washington v. Walter Harper*), the justices declared that a state prison can administer mind-altering drugs to a mentally ill inmate without his or her consent, merely on the professional say-so of doctors. The Court ruled that prisons don't have to have consent in all such treatments as long as they are not considered "experimental." The Court *did* imply that if such drugs are used in a prison to control or punish an inmate instead of to provide necessary medical care, the Constitution might forbid it, and it affirmed for the first time a constitutional right to refuse forced drugging by government agencies if the drugs could change the chemical balance of a mind, cause severe side effects, or lead to death. But what stands out is that the prisoner in this case, Walter Harper—because he posed a danger to himself, others, and property—could be drugged against his will. In its decision, the Court upheld Washington State's procedure for doing so: a review of a decision to force the drugs on the inmate by a panel not directly involved in the inmate's care.

Michael Shapiro, a lawyer, bioethicist, and world authority on medicine and the law, believes that *Harper* has "changed a lot of things" because it addressed the due process issue involved in the so-called right not to be treated—and the outcome does not wholly favor the person society wants to treat. Shapiro explains, "To find out if someone has a procedural, or due process right, the Supreme Court must often decide if there is any underlying substantive or 'liberty' right, such as the right to die in the Nancy Cruzan case or the right not to be treated in the Harper case."

In the Cruzan case, the state court in Missouri found that although the family's procedural rights—to cut off their comatose daughter's life support—could be limited and that the state had a substantive liberty right to force treatment of Nancy, there was and is a fundamental right to die. By contrast, in *Harper*, the Court said that whatever Harper's liberty interest might be in being free of psychotropic drugs, it was not necessary to require a court review and extensive procedural setup to guarantee him due process. In effect, the Court said there is *no* fundamental right to be free of chemical invasions of one's mind; fortunately the Court did not go quite so far as to deny the right to refuse treatment. The impact of the *Harper* decision on psychosurgery performed on prisoners or violent inmates in hospitals is unclear and untested, but it could be interpreted to suggest that institutions have a right to impose certain treatments—as long as they are not experimental—on inmates or prisoners, without their consent if doing so would be in their and society's interests.

A second Supreme Court case that could have a bearing on

psychosurgery as a means of social control was cited in the *Harper* decision. Known as *Youngbird,* the case involved a prison's plans to target a severely mentally ill inmate for rehabilitation treatment that had no guarantee of success. As Shapiro explained,

> The Supreme Court said the inmate does have an important liberty interest—if not a fundamental right—not to be treated, but decided that the standard of review for that inmate's right is simply to defer to what the professional judgment is. What it says, basically, is that unless you can show that the professionals involved were all drunk or something or operating under a conflict of interest or not doing their job at all, then whatever they say, essentially, goes. All the reins are off. It's hard to believe but that's what it is.

Advocates of psychosurgery for violent and other criminal behavior take heart from such cases, particularly because the Supreme Court has a tendency, says Shapiro, "to keep its hands off the decision-making process in institutions," especially prisons. "There are lots of cases where there are important rights at stake, but as soon as they're involved in an institution, the military, or the like, the Court essentially says, 'Do what you want.' In the years before *Harper,* the overwhelming majority of state courts recognized the more powerful rights to procedural protections." Yale law professor Burt agrees. "My view today is that unless you're dealing with experimental treatments, it is easy to devalue prisoners and to use them as guinea pigs. These people have always been treated as expendable, and I think that's the way it's always going to be. They're scary people, they've done terrible things, and it's easy to let doctors claim authority over them." Some surgeons and psychiatrists, however, believe psychosurgery for violent behavior benefits patients at least as much as society, and possibly more.

"I'd like to see amygdalotomies or other operations for patients who are incapable of living in our society because of severe, violent behavior since their youth, people who are violent sociopaths, self-destructive, and will never get better and who will need to be watched all their lives," says California neurosurgeon Oscar Sugar.

"If these individuals who are a terrible problem to society come forward and volunteer, or who don't want drugs to dull them and who want to stop hurting themselves and others, we should be able to accommodate them."

The kind of patient he has in mind, he says, is James Edward Plough. In June 1990, apparently distraught over the repossession of his car, Plough walked into a finance office in Jacksonville, Florida, and killed eight and wounded five before killing himself in a spree of violence. Police said Plough was the same man who gunned down a man and woman on the street 33 hours earlier and that the 42-year-old laborer had been convicted of aggravated assault in 1971. If "Plough had been operated on 20 years earlier, he would have still needed surveillance and care, but both he and society would have been free of his unpredictable and violent outbursts," Sugar says.

Some psychiatrists, notably in Britain, say they support the need for research into neurosurgical treatment of some violent individuals. "I think it's perfectly reasonable as a subject of study," says Paul Bridges. "We've sent three such individuals to [operations] in the last 10 years and their results were extremely good. These were very violent people. The problem with developing psychosurgery for violence and this type of thing is that in America, you bungled it. You were always overdoing things."

Arrayed against those who propose even cautious, limited use of operations to treat aggression are those who still portray psychosurgery as a plot to control antiestablishment views or behavior. Psychiatrists and the law enforcement community may argue society's rights to safety, but the opposition says the price is too high. Psychiatrist Peter Breggin, for instance, insists that the medical profession could not and would not restrain itself unless the procedures are banned outright. With personal attacks on such proponents of psychosurgery as Tom Ballantine, William Sweet, and especially Vernon Mark and Frank Ervin, Breggin has argued that "there is a still greater political menace in the psychosurgery movement—the danger that all of our citizens will become potential victims as the nation is turned into one large therapeutic state dominated by technological totalitarians."

What Breggin and his supporters don't say, however, is that the violent patients who are the usual suggested targets of psychosurgery are also mentally ill. They are not ordinary criminals who lack a social conscience, nor are they political dissidents. And those who advocate psychosurgery on a limited basis are not suggesting a return of lobotomies. While Breggin and psychologist Stephen Chorover, also a zealous critic of psychosurgery, acknowledge that the classic prefrontal lobotomies are not the issue or the worry, they fear that whatever operation *is* used will be abused. They point out that many of the operations done long after the Walter Freeman era were still done inappropriately for everything from homosexual tendencies and frigidity to anxiety, schizophrenia, alcohol addiction, and delusions. In Mississippi, they say, Orlando J. Andy used psychosurgery on children who were hyperactive. In a 1974 article published in *Psychology Today*, Chorover estimated that 500 to 700 Americans underwent brain surgery to control behavior, not illness, and noted that no one in the United States is charged with keeping track of how much psychosurgery is done, to say nothing of following up on consent procedures, outcomes, and protection of subjects.

In 1986, in the *Journal of Hospital and Community Psychiatry*, Leonard Roy Frank carried on the Breggin-Chorover tradition, claiming that American psychiatry is a political movement that oppresses patients. It's not a medical specialty, he wrote, but an instrument for the social control of people whose ideas, actions, and way of life "threaten or disrupt established power relationships within families, communities, or society." Psychiatry's "instruments," he wrote, are involuntary incarceration and "so-called treatment in facilities in which inmates are brutalized, harassed, neglected, and humiliated. And the major somatic psychiatric treatments—drugs, electroconvulsive therapy, and lobotomy—have produced an epidemic of neurological and brain dysfunction, such as tardive dyskinesia associated with neuroleptic drugs and memory impairment associated with ECT."

Frank, who says his "psychiatric inmates liberation movement" (he's cofounder of the Network Against Psychiatric Assault in Berkeley, California) is a former psychiatric patient who claims he was abused and his civil rights compromised. He said he had been electroshocked so often that he had memory loss, learning disability, apathy, loss of creativity, pain, fear, and humiliation. "Tragically enough," he writes "psychiatrists still subject people to lobotomy and other psychosurgical techniques. And they're proud of it." He lambasted the American Psychiatric Association (APA) for publishing a report of the success of "modified lobotomy" (actually, cingulotomy) for intractable obsessional neurosis and charged the APA with opposing "every legitimate effort to establish and protect the human rights of those labeled mentally ill."

Responding to Frank's charges, Harvey Ruben, M.D., associate professor of clinical psychiatry at Yale University and vice-chairman of the joint commission on public affairs of the APA, acknowledged that "as long as psychiatrists are human, there will be episodes of unethical psychiatric practice and ineffective, sometimes damaging psychiatric treatment." But calling these incidents exceptions to the integrity of the profession and "the reality of mental illness," he defended the need for involuntary treatment and suggested that "controversies surrounding involuntary treatment are essentially social, legal, and legislative issues in which psychiatry has found itself in the middle."

As the twenty-first century nears, psychiatrists and others who treat the mentally ill are still in the middle and society's institutions are often in a muddle:

- In the 1970s, Oregon and California passed laws establishing psychosurgery review committees, which resulted in making both voluntary and involuntary procedures virtually impossible to perform. These laws have not been seriously challenged in court, however. Other states have not followed suit.

- In 1977, the U.S. National Commission for the Protection of Human Subjects of Biomedical and Behavioral Research recommended a national psychosurgery advisory board to pass on psychosurgery proposals from willing patients and also recommended that all hospitals have institutional review boards to be certain informed consent had been given. Yet the commission did not advise against psychosurgery even for involuntary patients, as long as they consented.

- In Canada in the 1970s, psychosurgery was banned for involuntary patients, and in Great Britain the Mental Health Act established a board that must pass on every psychosurgical procedure. But bills introduced in Congress to ban psychosurgery in the United States failed as did a proposal by Senator Edward M. Kennedy calling for establishment of a commission to study the operations.

- In 1979, Mark, Ervin, and Sweet gave up their psychosurgical practice and advocacy principally because of a cutoff in federal funding for violence research and a $2 million lawsuit brought by a patient whose family said his personality had been destroyed. The doctors were found innocent; the validity of their work was not successfully challenged. At the end of the day, the medical and psychiatric communities are essentially—again and still—left to police themselves.

In the past decade, what this has meant is a an occasional brush with Erickson's extremism and large-scale, deliberate disinterest in psychosurgery. Neither approach serves science or patients. As we'll see in the next chapter, careful pursuit of surgical solutions can give hope, but too much caution has a price.

CHAPTER EIGHT

MATTHEW

I must tell you that I am very afraid of this man. Even under guard he is unpredictable, very scary. He ... is like a feral animal, a cat. He raises his arms and dives into people. He could kill.

—MATTHEW'S NEUROSURGEON, 1990

The story of Matthew frames much of the reasonable and unreasonable debate over the need for psychosurgery and its potential abuse. Matthew has a social history of the kind of violent behavior Colorado's Dale Erickson would crush with exploitative psychosurgery and a medical history that makes modern psychosurgery a last—and long delayed—hope. The following excerpts from a letter written on January 4, 1990, to Matthew's lawyer from a neurologist describes the cold, clinical details:

... Matthew is a 24-year-old right-handed man who has had severe and uncontrollable seizures since age 11. The cause of the seizures is encephalitis, which is an infection [presumed viral] of the brain. This infection produced scarring which resulted in spontaneously recurrent abnormal electrical discharges. When the electrical discharges build up to a certain level he will have seizures. During his seizures, he will have an aura [warning] of an unpleasant emotion, he will become confused, he will yell, grimace, turn his [head] side to side and will run about.

I have personally observed several of these episodes. He appears very frightening to others during the episodes. On one occasion we had a laboratory technician hide behind the door for many minutes after Matthew slammed into the door during a seizure. If someone is in his path, he will stare at them, then run into them or push them violently out of the way.

We monitored him in our critical care neurology unit with video-electroencephalography recordings in June of 1986. During that time we could observe his typical rage episodes, and correlate them with abnormal electrical activity in the brain. His seizures have occurred as often as ten times a day.

On October 5, 1987, Matthew had surgery on the right side of his brain and on November 24, 1987 on the left side of his brain in a structure called the amygdala. This is a structure which is often involved in seizures and in manifestations of violent behavior.... Unfortunately, the procedure was of no lasting benefit to Matthew.... I believe that Matthew has sufficient brain injury that he cannot control his outbursts of aggression. Some of these are explicitly because of seizures, [and] completely beyond his control. Others are not related to seizures, but occur because he has brain damage, delusional thinking, and lacks the normal inhibitory behavior that people must exert in society. Regrettably, this is likely to be a continuing condition with Matthew.

It is sometimes difficult to tell whether violence is part of a seizure, or whether it is an acting out of "bad temper." In Matthew's case, I think all of these are [beyond his control.]... I am enclosing an article ... on Epilepsy and Violence: Medical and Legal Issues, for your review of these subjects.

Matthew's medical situation is unfortunate.... We have been unable to manage this satisfactorily with medications and with surgery ... I would hope that the court and authorities would view his problems as a medical rather than a criminal issue.

Matthew is slight in build with boyishly silky, slightly long, dark wavy hair, freshly barbered. He sports a neatly trimmed beard. On an early June evening, in 1990, he has permission for a "special" visit with his parents and a guest, special because authorities at the high-security hospital for the criminally insane are strict about the 19.5 hours allotted for visits to each inmate each week. Matthew has spent almost a year here and 16 more years in schools and hospitals for young people with severe neurologic and psychiatric disease. As the summer began, the internal review board at a prestigious medical center considered his parents' request for neurosurgery to get him out.

We had put our belongings in a metal locker behind the guard's desk, keeping only a small tape recorder, and passed through an airport-style metal detector. Armed guards escorted us through two sets of locked doors, along a corridor into a room with brown Formica furniture upholstered in bright blue vinyl. Matthew sits in one of the chairs—facing us—wearing khakis, clean white socks, blue slip-on Keds, a hospital shirt tucked neatly into his beltless pants, and sunglasses. A burly security guard stays for the visit, too—protection against Matthew's unpredictable and violent rages.

MATTHEW: (*Shaking hands.*) How do you do ma'am. How about a sound check? Sure. (*Leaning forward, singing into the tape recorder*) I just called to say I loooo-ve you, I just called to say how much I care.

VISITOR: I want to ask you about your feelings, Matthew, about getting a brain operation.

MATTHEW: Yes. I want to leave here. With violent seizures, I have been put here. They don't really know about them, and they think it's just me being bad and acting out. When I was in [a state mental hospital] this lady named Fran told me I was a bad case and making it up. Yes ma'am, she said it. But I'm not.

VISITOR: If doctors said to you, "Matthew there's a chance this could help," you would do this, have an operation on your brain?

MATTHEW: Yes. (*Turning to look at the guard talking loudly on a wall phone.*) Can you wait until he is off the phone? I am having trouble concentrating. I'm sorry for the interruption. Please excuse me for saying to wait.

VISITOR: When you have your violent seizures, do you remember anything?

MATTHEW: No—wait, wait, yes. Sometimes. Yeah. Like I was telling my father last night. I don't know how I do it. But—put your fingers over your ear (*we all cup our hands over our ears*) and for about a second, I hear a muffling sound. You can hear air coming.

VISITOR: You mean like putting a seashell over your ear?

MATTHEW: Yes, yes, yes, exactly, exactly. After that, I get a ringing sound in both ears. One time with a violent seizure, I was in the shower room up at ward eight, and I went into one of [the showers] and I went in there and I was hearing the ringing sound. I walked out and walked around in circles and I forget the man's name—not because of the seizure but I just forget—he opened the curtain and he was nude and he told me (*Matthew whispers*), "Touch my penis, touch my penis," and I touched it, and I remember this during the seizure. And what happened was this man Rudolph ...

VISITOR: A person who works in the hospital?

MATTHEW: Yeah, and he walked in and I hit him—I forget where—I hit him and he grabbed me, and I think we were fighting. (*Matthew clenches his fists and works them back and forth to indicate a fight.*) And he threw me in seclusion, and it's just that I think some of this problem, fifty-fifty, is, you know, part of violent seizures and they [the attendants] just ... just ... (*a long pause*).

VISITOR: They don't know what to do?

MATTHEW: They don't know if it's a seizure or ... if like once when I was on [ward] three I just want my way. Wanting your way, what I mean by that is, on three, here I am, and I was mad and when I get mad, first I'm mad, then I'm madder, then madder and madder and so forth. [But] on eight I wasn't about to blow my top or get mad.

MATTHEW'S MOTHER: Or get out of control?

MATTHEW: (*Smiling and with a chuckle.*) Yes, thank you, out of control. What happened was, they said, "Matthew, how long would you like to be in your room?" [I guess all the] seclusion rooms were taken or something, I'm not sure. So they put me in my room and I was laying down like this (*he leans over in the chair onto his side*) and suddenly I went into a seizure like that (*he snaps his fingers*) and with no ringing in the ear or anything.

VISITOR: Sometimes you have a warning and can remember and sometimes you can't.

MATTHEW: Yes ma'am. And what happened was I was laying on my bed and I guess I got scared or something else bad and I grabbed the pillow and put it over my face and I started to scream and after that, well, I forget what happened but nothing positive. I went to a screened window in the room and I was banging on that, and screaming, not from the seizure but just screaming and a lady walked in and said, "Matthew, if you don't stop it I'll take your cigarettes away from you." And so I'm in this seizure.

MATTHEW'S FATHER: No, you said you were not in the seizure. That you are finished with the seizure. Did this happen after the seizure? Can you tell when the seizure is over? That's what you told me before. Your mind is fuzzy and you don't always know what's going on.

MATTHEW'S MOTHER: Can you feel when it's over?

MATTHEW: Sometimes I can. Sometimes I'm not really conscious. This one I'm talking about was one where I was still in seizure. I will say that when I went to the [screened-in] window, I was banging with my hand and banged on two beds, and what happened is that I had a feeling like one time that I was looking through this window on three and so I … (*long pause*). I couldn't control what I was doing, but my mind was telling me what to do. Like I … if I was in seizure now I'd look at this wall (*he points to a wall next to us*) and say let's do that and I would go to the wall and kick it or whatever, and that's what it was like at the screened window and I saw that, and I thought of things.

VISITOR: What things?

MATTHEW: (*Glancing quickly at his parents.*) My mother and father know about this. About God. What it is, is that I had a feeling that this happened before, that I'd, that I did that before and, well, what it was then was there was this other window and this man would always tell me to look out the window. He said, "Matthew look what's out there," and I'd say "What, what," and ... once he said to me, "Matthew look out there, look at that," and I said, "No, no I'm not about to look out there because it will happen again."

VISITOR: What happened then that you did not want to happen again?

MATTHEW: I'm not about for that to happen again.... What it was, I had this feeling that the person said to me, "You'll see out the window, you'll see what happens when you die." And so I um, I just had the feeling I was supposed to do this and do that, and I was in the seizure but for some reason I ... well ... like what I said about the wall.

MATTHEW'S MOTHER: Is this the thing where you believed God was out there, out of heaven, and it was your fault that God wasn't in heaven anymore and that's why so many terrible things were happening to you and everyone else and—

MATTHEW: Yes. Also, I had a feeling I was supposed to bang the window and beds, and I was there and I hit the window like this (*he demonstrates with his arm*) and [a] male staff [member] was called and he said, "Matthew, calm down now," and they put me in bed and next thing I knew, they shut the door and took my clothes off.

MATTHEW'S FATHER: We've heard this story before; it's going on too long.

MATTHEW: (*To his mother.*) I'm sorry I interrupted you before.

VISITOR: What makes you happy?

MATTHEW: Music. Mostly Beatles.

VISITOR: What is your favorite?

MATTHEW: Uh. "Sergeant Pepper's Lonely Hearts Club Band." And songs on their first album. My brother taped it for me. Mostly what I like to do is (*turns to his mother*) ... tell her what I liked to do, what that girl at the wedding.... Dance. Yes.

VISITOR: Your mother showed me the picture of you dancing at your brother's wedding.

MATTHEW: The other day I made up a new step where you jump up and then do this (*he slaps his thighs*).

MATTHEW'S MOTHER: I'm always amazed that you can remember words to songs and dance steps, but not your numbers or sometimes the alphabet or days of the week. That's your brain, the part of it that is healing.

VISITOR: If you could leave here, what would you like to do?

MATTHEW: You mean a job?

VISITOR: Anything.

MATTHEW: I would like to go home with my parents and see my sister-in-laws, my brothers, and my neighbors. And my grandmother. Whenever I get to two months without acting out, I act out or get a bad seizure, and then I have to start over and I can't go home ... (*long pause*). I'm trying to explain *why* I do things, not just what I do. Now this guy John [an inmate], he and I had an argument, he spit in my face, going down stairs. We were walking and my foot slipped on, and I lost my balance, and my hand was on the rail and instead of falling and busting my head open, I put my hand out so I would only break my arm (*he laughs*). Which would you like to do more? Anyway, John was in front of me and I accidentally pushed him, and what happened is, everybody saw that and thought I was pushing him and so when we got downstairs, he hit me with a plastic juice container and then he was slapping me or something and somehow he was off of me and I kicked him.... I got put in seclusion, and he got put in seclusion, and I don't think that was fair.

VISITOR: What wasn't fair?

MATTHEW: I'm getting tired of staff members keeping on me every time I was moved to a new ward. Every time, they'd say [it would be] two months [of good behavior] before I could go home and then (*turning to his father*) remember when I told this guy who could not pronounce my last name and I said, "Call me Pollack, nigger" (*laughter from the black security guard*) and he walked to me and so what it was, the staff got angry.

MATTHEW'S MOTHER: Did you admit that you shouldn't have said it? That it was wrong?

MATTHEW: No, because remember this one guy I knew and he was a friend and he was black and we called each other those names. I didn't mind, a word's a word. But I have to stay here longer when this happens, because one of the staff members keeps on me. One thing on my mind is to have a job. But I like the things my father and I used to do. We went to [a] park and walked around a lot. I'd like to live in a group with other people, and the Epilepsy Foundation has places, and that's where I'd like to go after I'm out of here, yes ma'am.

MATTHEW'S MOTHER: You forgot someone else you want to visit when you leave here.

MATTHEW: (*Smiling broadly.*) Yes. Jonathan [an infant nephew].

VISITOR: Is it okay with you if I come to the hospital and see you when you come for surgery?

MATTHEW: Yes, ma'am. Yes, even just to talk or just to visit.

VISITOR: I've talked to your doctor about you. It was okay with him and your parents. But it has to be okay with you, too.

MATTHEW: He's [the surgeon] a nice man. But what he did to my hair last time wasn't (*laughter*). He shaved it here and there and then the shaver didn't work! I looked like Kojak.

MATTHEW'S MOTHER: I said to [the surgeon], "Thank God you're a neurosurgeon because if you were a barber you'd be out of business!"

MATTHEW'S FATHER: Matthew always thought on those walks in the park that if he couldn't be a lawyer or a computer expert like his brothers, he had to be a garbage man. But there's a lot in between.

MATTHEW: I'd like to be an electrician.

MATTHEW'S MOTHER: What about horticulture? When you were planting things at that one hospital, you did that really well.

MATTHEW: Yeah.

MATTHEW'S MOTHER: Remember how many times we talked about some things you can't be? Like an airline pilot? But there were a heck of a lot of things you can be?

MATTHEW: That's one thing that gets me very angry about epilepsy, about my brain. Like I can't be a truck driver or do that. And (*he's makes an angry face*), yes, I'm angry because before the viral encephalitis and the epilepsy ... (*he pauses and thrusts his right hand with index finger extended into the air*) it was "Dr. Matthew!"

MATTHEW'S MOTHER: He'd have done it, too, no question. He'd have been a doctor. He talked about it from the time he was little boy, up to the minute he got sick when he was ten.

MATTHEW'S FATHER: After he got the encephalitis, everything left. Matthew didn't remember knowing how to count or to say the alphabet or even how to walk for a long time. Now he can do some things.

MATTHEW'S MOTHER: His brain is healing. Once you couldn't walk, do you remember that?

MATTHEW: I used to be very good at, what was it ... spelling. Every time there was a spelling bee, they would say to some guy, "How do you spell cat?" and he'd say, "K-a-t" and then they'd ask me, and I'd say, "C-a-t." I was the best in that. And also capitals of ... (*long pause*).

MATTHEW'S MOTHER: States?

MATTHEW: Yes. States. In that I wasn't the best, but pretty good.

MATTHEW'S MOTHER: He was always happy, too. That was lost, too. He liked being Matthew.

VISITOR: Things aren't fair, are they?

MATTHEW: No, not fair.

VISITOR: What will you do after we leave tonight?

MATTHEW: I'll get in pajamas. The females take showers tonight, then we sit around, watch TV—"Star Trek" maybe. We can smoke and do canteen.

MATTHEW'S MOTHER: Your neck is bleeding, Matthew. Is that the cyst they lanced? (*She gets up, dabs at it with a handkerchief. She sees it is not serious and gently ruffles his hair.*) Are you going to bed early to save cigarettes? Conserve them? Don't you have enough?

MATTHEW: (*Explaining to the visitor.*) We're only allowed one pack a day of cigarettes, so what I do, I go to bed eight thirty or nine after canteen snacks. I have a friend, Curt, and Leonard on my ward and Curt (I call him dumbfart and he calls me Mattfart), and he goes to canteen for me.

MATTHEW'S FATHER: Matt you're a survivor. Don't forget that.

MATTHEW: They say I don't belong here. Patients say it. Ray, he says, you don't belong here.

MATTHEW'S MOTHER: What does mommy say. I say it. You don't belong here.

MATTHEW: I will get out if I can stay calm, cool, and collected. (*Lots of laughter.*)

The hour is over. Matthew shakes hands. The guard asks another to escort the visitors out so he can take Matthew back to his ward. Matthew is smiling in the hall. He extends his arms out wide and says something to the visitor in Polish. His father translates: "He says he loves you, and will you marry him?"

Matthew's parents live in a middle-class neighborhood in a medium-size, Mid-Atlantic city. His father, retired after a nearly fatal heart attack several years ago; he had worked in a maritime industry plant as an engineer. His mother, robust and sad, is a full-time homemaker. Their superclean brick row house is pleasantly furnished and crowded with memorabilia of their children's childhoods, but their memories are overwhelmed by the details of Matthew's sickness, which began with a viral illness during a vacation at the beach when he was ten.

MATTHEW'S MOTHER: The first really awful time was after his initial illness, after we thought he might really get completely well. I'll never forget it. Matt came out of the bedroom shrieking that his hands were growing, that he had to go to the bathroom, but the "poopie" was all over and was attached to him by strings and begging us to cut them. We thought he was having a nightmare. So, his daddy went to lay down with him and as soon as he finally fell asleep—Jesus, it was two in the morning—his dad came back to bed with me. Then at eight A.M. we heard Matthew [again]. We heard him running. He was only a little boy. It was his first *grand mal* seizure, and it left him delusional, hallucinating, robotlike, and walking into walls. He stopped breathing.... we headed for the hospital.... That's when his hospitalizations became multiple and the specialists diagnosed him as having brain damage from a viral infection. That's what they think, though they'll never really know, and the seizures began in earnest, one after the other, sometimes hundreds a day and violent.

MATTHEW'S FATHER: He was like an animal, as strong as a bull, even at that young age so many years ago. He'd bite, pull out his mother's hair, put his arm through glass, throw furniture, all accompanied by horrible screaming. He was never aware of any of this, of course, and even today, at 25, he has no memory of that entire summer and fall.

MATTHEW'S MOTHER: Drugs worked for a while, and he'd come home from the hospital and start school again. We sent all our kids to parochial school, because they had strict discipline and good classes and the sisters, the nuns, really took an interest in them. Matt wanted to be a doctor, from the time he was little. I kept thinking that he was not the family scholar, so how would he do it? But I never really doubted that he would.

MATTHEW'S FATHER: We had to make sure he was restrained on the number of occasions that he was hospitalized. He would bite his mother's ear. And he would make these inhuman noises. If he ever got a hold on you, he'd grab you like a vice.

MATTHEW'S MOTHER: It's a helplessness you feel every day of Matthew's life. Among other things, it took more than a year for doctors at [the medical center] to finally witness one of the animal rages we were living with and fearing every day. You know, like when you stop having a toothache when you go to the dentist. He wouldn't have them when we went to the hospital or for checkups and it got to a point where no one believed us. Our credibility was at stake. We were accused of being hysterical, of exaggerating, of not wanting to care for Matthew.

MATTHEW'S FATHER: Well, I guess we had the last word on that. Sometimes I'm glad it happened the way it did, when Matt had this really bad seizure attack. There are still doctors there who won't be alone in a room with him. Who can blame them? They even got it on videotape.

MATTHEW'S MOTHER: A lot of good it did Matthew. It came too late. Remember, hon, when he first was sick and the nurses who refused to restrain him when we warned them? We were sent home for a night's sleep and that child threw himself out of bed and badly injured his already fragile brain. And those damn clerks who endlessly insisted on taking more long histories each time we brought Matthew into the emergency room. I couldn't believe it. There were files ten miles long on him already and we had to tell the same stories and histories over and over. Once, he turned over our dining room table. We'd be eating, calm, happy, everyone enjoying the dinner and then suddenly, we'd hear "Uuunnnnnnhh-hh!!!!!! unhhhhhhhhhHHHHH!" and growling. And I'd say, "Matthew, Matthew look it's mommy, it's daddy, you're home, it's okay," but he wouldn't know where he was. And for a long time doctors and therapists would tell us that he was a behavior problem, that he *could* control the behavior. Sometimes I believed it. Sometimes I wanted to believe it. But we were living with this. We knew damn well he couldn't.

MATTHEW'S FATHER: One day we went to the seizure clinic for blood tests of his drug levels and we were in the courtyard to smoke and he began to attack me with animal noises, and he burst through the security guards and raced through the seizure clinic. Two doctors grabbed him. He growled and fought. He ripped their clothes. They got a real eyeful. He was well over 18 by then. When this happened, the doctor said to bring him into the intensive care unit to monitor him. They strapped him down, and he just tore the cloth strips off. He made huge screams. That was when they videotaped him. It comes from nowhere, out of the blue. You can't predict it. Until this incident, the older doctors especially couldn't understand why he needed to be restrained. No one believed us until he broke through the straps and turned his hospital bed upside down and shrieked and shrieked. His mother went into the room to try to calm him. She took her life in her hands. But the window was opened. Matthew was at the window. He could well have thrown himself out. Within two hours, there were locks on those windows.

MATTHEW'S MOTHER: Well, now he is in a hospital for the criminally insane, but he is not a criminal really, and whether or not he is psychotic is open to question. We know the things he does are bad. But his brain is damaged, and no one can predict when he'll get his attacks. And he is a real pain with his compulsions. Sometimes, he gets depressed and obsessed with anything he hears, sees, or talks about for long periods of time. We can't tell him about an upcoming event, even a happy one, like when his brother was getting married. He'll just obsess about it, never let go, never stop asking when, when, when until it happens. It's unbearable for him and for everyone around him.

MATTHEW'S FATHER: I visit him every day they let me, every day.

MATTHEW'S MOTHER: I don't know how he stands it, how he does it. I can't visit that way anymore.

MATTHEW'S FATHER: You know why. You love him as much as I do, but you don't want to fight everything out there. I go there to see him, but I also go there because if I didn't, they'd, well, they might not do what all they're supposed to do. Some places were better for Matthew. This place can be cruel. I don't mean that they mean to hurt him, but they do. Sometimes on purpose and sometimes not, and I'm not going to let it go by.

MATTHEW'S MOTHER: God, we're hated everywhere, by every institution he's ever been in, and there have been a lot. We're aggressive in demanding rights for him, and we have a lawyer in the family, Matt's brother.

MATTHEW'S FATHER: Yeah, but it's a catch-22. If we fight for his rights, he could get punished by the staff if we win one for him. If we don't fight, he loses anyway. Like the cigarette business is typical.

MATTHEW'S MOTHER: I don't like it that he smokes. I wish we wouldn't encourage it. But I guess that's not the point.

MATTHEW'S FATHER: No. Matt's allowed a few cigarettes after every meal and he's an addicted smoker. It's one of his few pleasures, but sometimes if he's violent, if he acts out, he is given extra medication and he sleeps through his meals and smoking period. Then he's not allowed to have them when he wakes up. They tell him he "missed" his smoking time as if it were his own fault and he should be punished. So then he has more rage attacks and they give him more drugs and the cycle begins all over again. He's where he is now because of threats on people and fights, and they say he attacked a nurse with a fork at a state mental hospital where he had been for many years. Well, they deny it but we really believe that some of the staff wanted him out of there because, technically, he was too old, and so this one nurse taunted him and provoked him.

MATTHEW'S MOTHER: The bottom line is that no one and no place wants Matthew. Sometimes, when he has all these delusions and terrors and doesn't even know who we are, he makes us tell him over and over who we are. At those times I don't want him, either. My worst nightmare then and now is that in a desperate need and search for affection, human contact, and love, he will be exploited, sexually and emotionally, by other inmates.

MATTHEW'S FATHER: He's already had one round of surgery to try and control his epilepsy. It didn't work. Now his doctors have some new techniques and there is a chance that more surgery could help. Even if we give consent, the doctors tell us that the ethics committee at the hospital might not approve it, because it's risky; he could be paralyzed, he could get worse, it might not work. They can always keep him heavily sedated until he finally gets sick and dies. But, my wife knows this, I want to have this chance for him. I believe he can still get better, if not well. Why not try?

MATTHEW'S MOTHER: Right now, I don't want that. I don't want to go through that again. We were so hopeful that last time. I really believed that it would make him better. Now I know that he'll never get better. The best we could hope for is that he'd get easier to manage. Or he could die, or get worse. This is so hard. I am so tired of talking about it.

MATTHEW'S FATHER: If he has the operation, and stops having rages for at least two months, he can leave the place he's in and go to another hospital or into a private one if we can get the insurance to pay for it. Matt's on Medicaid. The finances are tricky. He gets Social Security disability of $438 a month, of which he gets to keep $35 and the rest goes to pay for his care in the hospital or institution at the rate of $12 a day. We give him one $135 a month for canteen, plus eyeglasses and personal items.

MATTHEW'S MOTHER: Matt can never completely take care of himself. I'm afraid to hope that more surgery can help him, maybe just enough so he can go into less-structured care, but also just enough that he might get scared or hurt himself or get hurt. I feel guilty about not going to see him very much. I'm worried about it. If we tell him to get his okay for us to come, then he'll drive himself and us nuts asking about it. And then he might get upset while you're there.... The Epilepsy Foundation has a group home. If he got better, they might be able to take him there, get him vocational training. I know that. In the institution, I worry about men taking advantage of him. And I worry about what will happen to Matt when we go. His brothers will take care of him. They're very close, but it hurts, and its tough. God it's tough. What is especially heartbreaking is that his anger is not bad, not wrong. Matt knows what he has lost.

Less clear is what he might gain from surgery. But on November 20, 1990, two days before Thanksgiving, he, his family, and his doctors get the chance to find out.

7:15 A.M.: In the wide corridor of the medical center's basement neuroradiology suite, Matthew waits on a gurney, held securely in four-point restraints. With him are his mother, father, older brother Jim, and a guard from a state mental hospital. In anticipation of his cingulotomy, he had been transferred from the high-security prison-style hospital, and there is hope that if the surgery succeeds, the halfway house, sheltered workshop training, and independence await. Matthew is nervous but cheerful, wrapped in pastel gowns, his feet and legs in vented stockings, IV line taped securely to his right arm. "I'm not getting my hopes up too high this time," his mother says, her eyes on Matthew.

"I am," his father says. Matthew is quiet.

Matthew's surgeon walks by in a three-piece suit he'll soon exchange for pale green scrubs. He stops for a minute to talk, holding on all the while to his briefcase. He pats Matthew's foot. "I'll see you soon," he says.

Matthew's family will not see their son for the next nine hours.

In 1937, Henrich Klüver and Paul Bucy removed the temporal lobes of a normal rhesus monkey, depriving the animal of its amygdala, hippocampus, hippocampal gyrus, and all adjacent structures of its limbic system, or emotional brain. The animal developed what came to be known as the Klüver-Bucy syndrome. Instead of its usual aggressive, somewhat nasty temperament, the monkey was placid, tame, easily handled, impossible to provoke. It also was uninhibited and displayed other abnormal, sometimes compulsive, sexual and eating behavior. Over the next 20 years, other experimenters found that the taming effect Klüver and Bucy produced would occur with the removal or lesioning of the amygdala alone. By contrast, placing small areas of damage in the front of the hypothalamus nucleus produced permanently ferocious animals, and because of the many nerve connections between the two structures, scientists concluded that the amygdala is controlled through the hypothalamic structure.

Since the 1940s and 1950s, neurosurgeons have removed areas of the amygdala and the temporal lobe to stop violent behavior, with variable success. In 1987, they operated on both the right and left amygdala in Matthew, whose temporal lobe epilepsy apparently damaged circuits involved in the hypothalamus and left him with an unpredictable, assaultive, dangerous, hair-trigger temper. He also suffers from obsessive thoughts and behavior. "I must tell you," the surgeon said, "that I am very afraid of this man. Even under guard he is totally unpredictable, very scary. He has rage seizures and is like a feral animal, a cat. He raises his arms and dives into people. He could kill.'"

The stereotactic amygdalotomies unfortunately did not work. "We would have had to remove both temporal lobes to take care of the damaged circuitry," one of his doctors said. "That would have produced Klüver-Bucy syndrome. No way. Destroying the brain," he said, "is a kind of death."

After three years, dozens of rage seizures, and a violent assault on a nurse, surgeons will try again to kill—by cutting out—a small part of Matthew's abnormal brain, about a square centimeter of it. He'll have a cingulotomy, an operation designed to dampen motivation, to calm. It is also performed for cancer pain that even narcotics can't help. "I did one on a bone cancer patient," said the surgeon. "Before the operation he cried in agony all day. After, he was completely relaxed. He read most of the time. He had no more suffering. He had no more emotions, either, nor was he capable of any real mental work. It was drastic. Like a lobotomy. Matthew's will not be that drastic."

Drastic or not, there is nothing left to try. "This kid's brain is totally out of control," says a child neurologist who consulted on Matthew's condition. "When the amygdalotomies failed, his own neurologist wept. He said he didn't know how to face the family. He cried, he really cried. There's nothing left now but high-security institutionalization and sedation to the point of near coma. The new surgery is a chance. It's a Hobson's choice for all of us," he added. "Even if it stops the violent rages, we don't know if it will stop the obsessive behavior."

The medical center's institutional review board and ethics committee approved Matthew's surgery in the fall of 1990 and the surgeon put him on the operating-room (OR) schedule for November 20.

Operating Suite 2 really is a suite, a collection of rooms. The largest of the rooms is the operating room itself, but unlike a conventional operating room, it houses a modern CT scanner, with its hollow, scooped bed and donut-shaped scanning apparatus. Five freestanding monitors are on site as well, to track drugs and vital signs. Behind the scanner, radiation technician Vincent Lerie and scrub nurse Gerry Beveringen set up three sterile tables for equipment. Most prominent alongside the usual scissors, knives, sutures, gauze pads, needles, and tubes are the Radiofrequency Lesion Generator and the stereotactic halo that guarantees millimeter-precise positioning of the brain probe and needle tip that the Lesion Generator will heat to 75°C. Over the next hours, Lerie will switch it on ten separate times to destroy ten tiny pieces of brain tissue in Matthew's cingulate gyrus (*gyrus* simply means a "hill"), deep in the frontal lobes beneath his cerebral cortex. The cingulum itself is part of the paired structures of the limbic system that straddle the brain's central artery and carry signal-making nerve fibers around the system, including the signals that trigger Matthew's rage-producing seizures. While the temporal amygdala of Matthew's brain are structurally "miles away" from the cingulum, the circuitry is interconnected with it and with nerves in the hypothalamus, the center of defense and attack reactions. Thus interfering in one part of the circuit interferes in others "upstream" or "downstream."

The operation to be performed on Matthew borrows heavily from work by Tom Ballantine in Boston and Geoffrey Knight and Desmond Kelly in Great Britain. Their published experience with thousands of patients will make today's effort as precise and safe and promising as possible. In a procedure much like the one developed by Ballantine at the Massachusetts General Hospital, the heated needle will create dead space to act as a "firebreak" in Matthew's brain and, it is hoped, will stop transmission of rage-triggering signals from the frontal lobes. The stereotactic equipment, which makes electrical lesions in the brain, eliminates the risk of "blind," freehand reaches into the limbic system by automatically lining up points on the computer-made topographic "map" of Matthew's brain with the same points, in three dimensions, in Matthew's brain itself. In this way, the CT road maps guide the surgical probes safely past areas of the cerebral cortex covered by blood vessels and controlling sensory and motor areas, including smell and sight and arm and leg movement, and safely away from the thalamus, which is the main relay station taking messages to the higher centers of the cortex.

To compare this cingulotomy to old prefrontal lobotomies or leukotomies is like comparing a Civil War conscript's musket fire target precision of a Tomahawk missile, or a child's first crayon drawing to an architect's precise blueprint. The lesions to be made in the "hill" in Matthew's cingulum are anatomically "miles" from the temporal lobe, but the changes—the calming, flattening—they produce will be somewhat similar. That's because the neural fiber pathways work in parallel and bundle together in various spots deep in the brain. Thousands of psychosurgeries, along with modern technology, have brought "less of the knife" and enough of the desired effect, without the mutilating damage of frontal lobotomy.

Space is crowded in the suite, especially with plans for half a dozen or more onlookers, among them radiologists, students, and physician assistants. Most of these will watch from behind a lead shield glass wall that isolates the operating room and its sterile environment from the computer tomography control room that has regular room air. The glass-walled anteroom faces the OR and contains four computer monitors and other equipment. All of it will be used to display and interpret scanner information and pinpoint targets for the team that planned this sortie into Matthew's limbic system with the precision of a military operation.

An adjacent small room holds the computer that operates the scanner, and connecting the areas is a small corridor and *cul de sac* enclosing a "light wall" to read the pictures made of the scans, a 30-cup, ever-filled coffee pot, telephones, desk, cartoon art, a refrigerator, and more monitors.

7:50 A.M.: Toby Eagle, the nurse anesthetist, and Steve Derrer, the anesthesiologist, bring Matthew in and transfer him to the CT scanner bed where he will stay, anesthetized, throughout the operation. They gently explain the tubes. "Matt asked a lot of questions when we talked earlier," says the anesthesiologist, who clearly loves his work. "God, it's the best. Sometimes I can't believe they pay me to do it."

He will spend the next eight hours keeping Matt's breathing rate steady (around 37 or 38 respirations per minute), his heart rate at about 67 or 68, and levels of drugs fed through tubes into his body at just the right balance for safety and effectiveness. Then he'll awaken him. "Matt, I'm going to give you some medicine through the tube," he says.

"It'll feel hot for a second," says Eagle. Matt whimpers for an instant and then he is quiet. Eagle puts a nose and mouth mask quickly over his face. "Just a little oxygen," she fibs to him. It's really nitrous oxide, and in just moments, Matt is asleep. Derrer has injected a cocktail of drugs through the tube—pentothal, fentanyl, fluorane. "Have a good rest, Matt," Eagle says gently. He can't hear her.

7:56 A.M.: Eagle passes a breathing tube into Matthew's throat, adds more lines. Beveringen inserts a Foley catheter to collect Matthew's urine. The front part of his long, silky hair is shaved from the front of his forehead to about halfway back. They leave the rest, including beard and sideburns. "He cares a lot about his hair," says Beveringen. "Most young guys do." Matthew's eyes are taped shut now and the supporting part of the stereotactic frame is placed under his head and shoulders, clamped to the bed that supports him and screwed into his skull with four white screws at the temples.

8:35 A.M.: Lerie clears everyone out of the room so he can turn on the CT scanner, which hums. The scanner takes a long series of X-ray "slices" of Matthew's brain, pictures that will give the surgeon and his helpers the coordinates to set the stereotactic frame's probe guide in exactly the right planes—back to front, side to side, and top to bottom—so that every lesion is made in the right spot. Surgeon Sumio Uematsu, the radiologists, the neurologists, and the technicians are crammed into the control room on and off for most of this first hour. Many will move in and out, back and forth between the sterile operating room and the control room. And for the first of many times, concentrating on the brain images, Uematsu "contaminates," breaking the sterile barriers of his gloves and gown. The nurses groan; they're used to regloving and gowning him. He doesn't care. He needs to point, check textbooks and drawings, make notes. At about 9 A.M., he's looking at reconstructed scans that highlight an important landmark: the telltale butterfly-shaped structure of the corpus callosum. From there, it's only about two centimeters back—down—to the cingulum, the target. He also locates, among the varied shades of white, gray, and black, the major anterior pericallosal cerebral artery he must avoid.

Dozens of scans are done, more than 35. "It's got to be right, perfect, absolutely right. We need to check and recheck, check and recheck," says Uematsu. He keeps saying this aloud, yet to himself, almost like a prayer, or a mantra.

9:30 A.M.: A neurologist who has cared for Matthew for many years arrives with a photocopy of a medical-journal article written by Ballantine. In it are detailed photographs of the sites in the brain where Ballantine recommends placing lesions. The neurologist refers to the lesions as "cuts," although they will be made by heat, not a knife. "Ballantine did more than 600 of these cingulotomies," he announces in the CT room. "Most of them were for chronic pain. This is different, of course."

Still holding the article, he gazes at Matthew's draped form through the glass wall. He does not go into the operating room, even when this first round of scanning is completed at 10:15. Instead, he leaves the suite to see Matthew's family. He will come and go often during the day.

10:16 A.M.: Physician's assistant Debbie Mandelblatt places a white stretch cap on Matthew's skull and over the cap, a clear, stretchable plastic, not unlike thick plastic kitchen wrap, and fastens it down like a sausage casing. The wrap holds the scalp skin taut and sterile and isolates the slits the surgeon will cut in it to reach the skull and brain. "We'll make two burr holes, or entries," Uematsu tells his assistants. "The right side first." Two hours and 15 minutes into this operation, the first real surgery is about to happen.

The monitors are clicking, instruments are readied. Beveringen is in place across from the surgeon. The masked Lerie is circulating, his ungloved hands appropriate for moving nonsterile equipment, centering overhead lights, checking supplies. Without discussion, he tapes a sheet of lined copybook paper—the kind from a child's notebook—on the wall to the right of Uematsu. Everyone in the room stares at it. It has the following handwritten on it in block print:

RIGHT
AP = +19
LAT = +13
VERT = 29

Uematsu, Mandelblatt, and Lerie study it especially carefully, glancing back at it dozens of times over the next 15 minutes. These are the target coordinates, "checked and rechecked," then copied down from the scores of reconstructed overlapping scanner images. These are the numbers that tell the surgeon precisely how deep, how far in, how far over, how far down to send his needles. And before he even puts the needles in, they tell him how to set the gauges on the stereotactic frame. It's a somewhat cumbersome affair. First, two people take the top part of the frame that will hold the needle probe in the proper position and place it over a tabletop mock-up of the half that is already attached to Matthew's skull.

This "double" or "phantom" of the so-called positioning platform frames not a brain, but a triangular base made of Plexiglas with steel dowels jutting up to fasten the top of the frame. The base also holds an adjustable vertical column in its center, an upright shaft with a tiny tip on it that represents the target, ground zero, in Matthew's brain. Using CT scan plotting charts (the coordinates are taken from the charts), the phantom frame is used to position the probe and lock it on the target before it is put in the real frame on the patient's head. The base is set to the coordinates from the plotting charts.

This stereotactic device is the modern descendent of an instrument first introduced in 1908 by Sir Victor Horsley and R.H. Clarke to study the relationships between brain structures and behavior by stimulating or surgically disconnecting specific areas of an animal's brain. Surgeons first used it on a patient in 1947.

The challenge then—as now—was to place current-carrying probes or needles deep under the cortex without damaging structures overlaying the target area. The solution was a way to tilt and rotate the probe at precise angles.

Using the phantom device, the surgical team first inserts an electrode into a "holder," or "carrier," arm of the frame and sets the tip of the target bar to the exact center of the target brain tissue, based on the plotting charts. The electrode is advanced to the computer-calculated distance until the electyrode tip just touches the target bar. Everything is sterile. The carrier is then rotated, tipped, and set to the surgeon's desired angle of entry, an angle set to bypass and avoid striking major vessels in the brain area. Coordinate setting is also done to guide the problem through all the planes of the brain: anterior-posterior (front to back); lateral (side to side); and ventrodorsal (top to bottom).

Five separate times they validate the settings on this mock-up before the coordinates are locked down. Now the electrode probe is positioned on every plane. It can be moved in any direction and the probe reaches to the target from any direction, and the target will always be in the center of the stereotactic frame.

10:30 A.M.: Uematsu makes a one-inch cut in the plastic wrap and skullcap, then slices the skin and underlayers of the scalp. He uses a retractor to hold the skin back and stitches it in place. It's quiet in the room as Uematsu picks up a hand drill, and drills the burr hole, beginning slowly and building to a vigorous circular motion with the handle. He drills and drills into the skull. With suction and irrigation, pieces of bone and tissue gush out on the table under Matthew's head, but very little blood. Matt sleeps peacefully.

10:45 A.M.: Drilling stops. Uematsu uses currettes, tiny sharp curved knives, to clean out the hole. The top half of the stereotactic frame is put over the hole. There is a faint smell of burning as he electrically seals or coagulates small blood vessels covering the brain. Then, it's time to set the electrode needle into the brain. The necessary apparatus, already locked into the right place, is lifted from the mock-up frame and placed over the bottom half of the device affixed to Matthew's skull.

The surgeon will not need to make any judgments about where to put it. The probe will go through the holder and stop automatically at the target point. He selects the right-size probe—an eight-inch-long needle really—from the stainless steel tray held by Beveringen and sets it aside. The frame is ready, the coordinates have been checked a dozen times.

"No," he says. "We'll scan again." Another cross-check. He will introduce the eight-inch needle into the target area, inject air (0.3 cubic centimeters) into the brain, take more scans, and make sure the probe will be within the targeted brain tissue in the cingulum.

Lerie clears the OR for the scans.

11:30 A.M.: It has taken 45 minutes and two injections of air to learn that the black dots of air highlighted in the scanning images are right on the target cingulum. "Better than textbook, better than perfect," Uematsu exclaims for the first of many times that day. "Now. Now, we're ready to go." Everyone files back into the OR. Uematsu is regloved and gowned; he had "contaminated" again.

The radio frequency heat-generated electrode probe is replaced by the needle tip so that it is resting on the target. Beveringen wheels over the Radiofrequency Lesion Generator, irreverently referred to as the "cooking machine." It is the only gallows humor of the day. But it is accurate. The electrode is hooked up to the source of current. Beveringen squirts a clear gel on a tinfoil-covered rigid plate and inserts it under Matthew's back. Then he runs a wire with an alligator clamp to the retractor handles and hooks it up. "Grounding Matthew," he says to no one in particular. "Grounded."

"In case something breaks," Uematsu explains.

11:43 A.M.: "Set for 75°C for 90 seconds," Uematsu orders Beveringen. The dials are set.

"Okay," Uematsu says. "Cook." He forces a smile. No one returns it.

Through the same hole, Uematsu positions the probe four more times in the same plane to create four other tiny lesions around this first central lesion. Some at 90 seconds, some at 45 seconds. All at 75°C. "Cook," he orders. "Cook," again. "Cook." "Cook." The lesions are less than an eighth of an inch apart, all on the right side. That's Matthew's right, his right hemisphere, his right cingulum.

While cooking occurs, every pair of eyes in the crowded space behind Matthew's head—without exception and for no really good reason—is fixed on the probe sticking out of the skull. No one can see the targets and won't until scans are done. It's close to noon. The right side is pronounced "finished." Lerie clears the room again for the scans that will confirm the lesions. There is not a chance they are *not* on target. Nevertheless, there is tension, waiting for the black and white and gray proof. If the lesions have been made, and in the right places, they will appear as tiny black blots over the computer-made cross-hairs etched into films made earlier in the morning.

The first scans are too shallow to detect any lesions. Suddenly, the reconstruction of the deeper scan of the target plane comes up. "There," says Uematsu quietly, pointing to a perfect circle of black blots. "All there. Perfect. Better than the textbook. Now, ready to do the left side."

12:15 A.M.: "Do you know how we learned how long to cook?" Uematsu asks as he makes the second burr hole. "Egg whites. We used raw egg whites, in 1967, in our first studies, to see how long and how hot a temperature we needed to change transparent raw egg whites into cooked opaque whites and to create a hole that would not close up by measuring the diameter of the cooked white area in the transparent egg white."

Lerie turns over the lined copybook paper, carefully peeling off the same piece of tape and retaping it to the wall on the reverse side. The frame's "double" is set for new coordinates:

LEFT
AP = +21
LAT = –9
VERT = –29

Over the next two hours, five more lesions are placed in the cingulum on the left side of Matthew's brain. The air target studies are again done to verify the placement, then they "cook," the heated tip cutting the brain. Then more scans make sure the lesions are sufficient and in place.

3:40 P.M.: Derrer has awakened Matthew and escorted him to the recovery room. Uematsu and others have talked to Matthew's family. "Perfect," Uematsu announces. "Better than the textbook." Then, they all must wait to see if the "textbook" surgery was not just successful in its execution, but also in its goal. Matthew's neurologist is nervous; he says there's much that can still go wrong, including brain damage or return of the seizures, which might have found an alternative pathway for the abnormal electrical signals.

6 P.M.: Matthew wakes fully and talks a blue streak, but then unexpectedly lapses into a stupor. He is apparently unable to talk, or move his limbs or arms. An angry, upset neurologist says "it's not looking good." They take Matthew back to the neuroradiology lab for an emergency scan. Everything looks okay. The doctors hope the problem is temporary, from swelling that will subside. Matt's parents are with him all night.

Wednesday, November 28, 11 A.M., eighth floor of the neuroscience wing: Matthew is propped up in bed in room 811, eating seedless red grapes from a plastic bag, half-watching a television set suspended from the corner of the ceiling above his bed. His mother is all smiles; his father grinning.

"God we are happy today," his mother says. "I knew it all the time. He's doing just great." Matthew has no pain, not even a headache, but he is still somewhat stunned and slow to react. Full recovery from the surgery is still days or more away, although he will go to a less-guarded psychiatric hospital on Sunday if all goes as planned. After six months without rages, they'll know if the cingulotomy has brought success, peace, and the chance for a better life.

That morning, little more than a week after his operation, Matthew remembers names and faces slowly, but he does remember. His arms and legs and toes work. He can talk. "Rodgers," he says after his mother's prompt of a visitor's first name. "Writing a book," he says. A moment later, there's a smile, which broadens when his father says quietly, "Perfect. So far perfect. Better than the textbook."

Over Memorial Day weekend 1991, six months after Matthew's surgery, his parents are still careful not to trumpet their hope. But all the signs remain positive. Over the holiday, Matt is spending most of his time on a home visit with his family, and weekend leave from the hospital is now regularly scheduled. Matt's social worker has begun the process of enrolling him in a special course at the hospital that teaches independent living skills—cooking fundamentals, washing clothes—because paperwork is under way to place him in a community-based group home.

"There have been no rages since his operation," Matt's mother says. "He's still having seizures but no rage episodes at all. And he seems to have much, much better control of his anger. It doesn't escalate into chaos. He takes the time to calm down when he becomes angry. We think we have a success here, but the doctors—and we—still don't know how long it will last. Six months, two years, twenty years. Who really knows? Our hospital hasn't had experience with this kind of case before."

The absence of experience is a lingering reminder of the ongoing ignorance surrounding the new psychosurgery, as well as the continuing political, medical, and social isolation of patients like

Matt and his family. Even without overt suppression of research and interest in surgical treatment of psychiatric and behavior disorders—even though there are pockets of interest among psychiatrists and neurosurgeons—there is still a giant wall of timidity that turns away heads and minds. The neurologist who has cared for Matt since he was 18 is leaving his post and the city to work elsewhere, taking from the community whatever limited expertise he developed and whatever influence and advocacy for the procedure he presented to his colleagues there. Yet even in the wake of success, the doctors don't want to "go public" with their endeavor. Lost in the silence is the fact that there are newer psychosurgical treatments for mental illness that need cheering on. So far, the cheerleaders are mostly the families of patients. And even their cheers are muted, reflecting the cautions and concerns of the medical profession.

Matt's mother says, "Matt's still scared. We are too. That suddenly something will happen. When Matt comes on visits, he gets angry with me at times because he senses that I'm still wary of being alone with him. If his daddy goes off briefly to the store and leaves me alone with Matt, I'm nervous. I'm still remembering those rages, his physical strength, how he could hurt others and himself. It hurts Matt now to think that I'm leery of him, that I'm afraid to be alone around him."

Confidence that the scars made in his brain can keep control of his mind will take time to build. Meanwhile, the family cautiously moves ahead. One of the community homes is only four blocks from Matt's family and the parents are divided about whether Matt should try for a bed in that one. His father says yes; his mother, no.

"Matt is used to having his daddy rescue him. He needs to learn to live on his own, to make it with other people," she says. "The social worker told us that if Matt is placed in a group home and gets frustrated or angry and leaves it for any reason, he won't be able to come back. If he's living so close to us, the temptation will be great to run home to daddy if things get tough. I don't think he should have that temptation. I think his dad is coming to my way of thinking about this, but we have to talk about it more."

They worry, too, about Matt's placement with mentally retarded men and women in the group home, because he is not retarded. But just as there are few medical centers ready, willing, and able to perform the surgery Matthew sought, so are there even fewer facilities to help assure his success in the aftermath.

Matthew's mother talks easily about his present and his near future, stopping only a moment to chase down her toddling grandson, for whom she's baby-sitting part of the holiday. "He keeps me running," she laughs. "He's learning to walk." Then her voice drifts off. "It's hot today," she says, "going to be in the nineties." No, she says in response to a question, they're not going to the beach on this holiday. "I think I'll stay in the air-conditioned house." Her thoughts, too, perhaps, are drifting, back to the summer holiday day 17 years ago, at the shore, when a young family watched their 10-year-old youngest son play in the heat of the day.

CHAPTER NINE

WHOSE MIND IS IT ANYWAY?
SOME QUESTIONS AND ANSWERS

Thinking is hard work. We don't want to have to think too hard about complicated things. So we make up rules that free us from having to make tough decisions.

—MICHAEL SHAPIRO, J.D., PROFESSOR OF LAW, UNIVERSITY OF SOUTHERN CALIFORNIA

Every act has consequences. The consequences of the 1960s and 1970s backlash against psychosurgery, for example, stopped practices that mutilated the brains of an estimated forty to fifty thousand Americans. It limited the potentially abusive power of psychiatrists and surgeons to experiment on hospital and prison inmates, and helped create a strong medical consumer movement and protection for mental patients. Other consequences were less predictable and less comforting. The backlash drove rational debate and research on psychosurgery underground and left a policy vacuum in the wake of the anger and hysteria. It hassled psychiatrists and neurosurgeons into abandoning operations not because they lacked compassion or skill, but because they worried more about public and professional opinion than the despair of their charges. The care of the mentally ill became a battleground for lawyers, families, politicians, and extremists with a giddy array of agendas. It almost completely cut off access to some proven, safe, and effective treatments, and produced great suffering.

In the drive to protect human subjects from any and all experiments, many are subjected to a pathetic quality of life in institutions and a fog of drugs. All but gone is any way to assess the risks and benefits of psychosurgery or address the ethical and moral issues that go along with altering the mind and brain. While the threat from the Dale Ericksons of the world is there, it is small; and there *are* patients, violent and otherwise, who might benefit from psychosurgery, who see it as a way out from behind prison bars or locked wards and are willing to take the risk. As long as the potential remains for psychiatric abuse of patients; as long as fear, uncertainty, and history haunt doctors and hospitals; as long as conflicting rights and responsibilities pose a tangle of possible decisions, the desire to avoid the hard job of thinking in favor of just saying no is understandable. But a refusal to grapple with the potential of modified psychosurgeries may be no better than the abuses of the past. Denying legitimate patients access to surgery may soothe the consciences of ethicists, psychiatrists, lawyers, and judges, but may be as abusive as Erickson's legislative proposals.

In obsessive-compulsive disorder like Susan's, was a decade of suicidal depression, drugs, and frustration a reasonable price to pay for help? What if she hadn't had an articulate lawyer-boyfriend and upper-class resources to take her to Britain? In the case of Matthew's violent rages, how long was long enough for him to languish with ineffective psychotherapy in a prisonlike asylum before a hospital was willing to give him a chance at getting out? His entire life is already so dominated by institutional psychiatry that he peppers his conversation with highly professional psycho-babble. How long was long enough for his family to anguish? To fight panic? To answer charges they "exaggerated" his condition to "get rid of" their son? To face hostility from insensitive nurses and hospital clerks fed up with Matthew's violence? To wear down bureaucrats who withheld financial aid they were entitled to until they threatened to sue for it? To plead with schools that held out hope then tossed out Matthew? To wait for hospital review boards that took years to meet and make decisions? "There's not a reason in the world anywhere to withhold this shot for him," one of Matthew's doctors told me when I inquired about the delay in going forward with his cingulotomy. "He's desperate and so are we. But he's not the owner of his own mind. The state, his parents, and the ethics committees are."

What's left for the mentally ill and those responsible for them? Can a balance be restored between the rights of patients to treatment and the obligation of society to protect the vulnerable? Or should we forget about it because the ethical dilemmas are too hard? As a popular film a few years ago about a quadripelegic's desire to die asked, to whom, indeed, does a person's "mind" and brain belong? Is our inability to truly know what is in another person's mind justification for the moral high ground of *never* tampering with it? Or is there some end point other than perfect safety and effectiveness by which to measure the outcome of treatment? Who can—and should—decide who gets a treatment and who does not? Who really has power over the modern tools of medicine and over patients' choices? Who wants the power? Who needs it? How do you get it?

Fortunately, there are psychiatrists, lawyers, ethicists, surgeons, and social scientists wrestling with these questions. During interviews with more than 40 of them, including a dozen whose careers have spanned the entire era of psychosurgery, many took the position that surgery for psychiatric illness would—and should—prevail, at least for small numbers of patients. Their goal is to find ways to resolve the thorny legal, social, and ethical issues and refrain from throwing the baby out with bath water. They will keep working at it, keeping in mind the object of their labor: the patients whose minds are at stake.

One who still labors at all this after almost four decades has a sign on his office door that proclaims, "Tiger Inside." Behind the door, there is one, with piercing eyes and ferocious energy. He is unapologetic about his chain smoking or his advocacy of psychosurgery. According to him, all psychiatrists fall into two categories: "ivory tower and red brick"; he hasn't much patience with the former. Even the recent death of his 48-year-old son in a car accident can't subdue the gutsy "cowboy" impression associated with both his Oklahoma heritage and his long career as a neurosurgeon at Harvard Medical School and the famed Massachusetts General Hospital.

For forty years, H. Thomas Ballantine stalked the medical jungle, becoming one of the nation's most vocal psychosurgeons until more political animals all but completely suppressed that part of his practice. Yet today, his name is synonymous with successful cingulotomy for obsessive-compulsive disorder and violent behavior; his publications are honored for their integrity and pored over by surgeons. Ballantine retired from the operating room three years ago, but still wears a straight pin in his lab coat lapel—the portable test instrument of choice among his crowd. And he keeps an aggressive stance with respect to "appropriate" surgery for psychiatric illness. "No one has the right to deny patients access to help," he says. "No one."

BALLANTINE: My interest in psychosurgery—how that word rankles some people—goes back to my days as an undergrad at Johns Hopkins. You know, in those days, and I don't know if it's true at present time, psychiatry was a subject for all four years of medical school, starting with a look into our own minds. We had to write autobiographical sketches. And there was Adolph Meyer, a very great and wonderful person, although he spoke from time to time in an almost unknown tongue as far as I was concerned. He had this heavy German accent.

I believe he coined the word *psychobiology* and he had on his staff a birdlike woman named Esther Richards who gave many lectures we *could* understand, and her point always was that you *never* make a psychiatric diagnosis unless you have absolutely ruled out an underlying medical one. What got through to me was the connection between the mental and the physical and I got interested in psychiatry. When I began my neurosurgical practice, I was doing a lot of disc surgery for bad backs and I extended my interest in the relationship between pain and depression. You see the treatment of chronic pain was often very helpful in treating clinical depression.

VISITOR: You did some lobotomies?

BALLANTINE: Yes, we called them leukotomies. I did a number of them at Maclean Hospital, not a lot, but some, with my senior associate. But I became disenchanted with that operation because of the side effects. But I was ambivalent. There was a more or less scientific study of use of leukotomy or lobotomy in VA hospitals after World War Two that compared the rate of discharge from the hospital of operated and nonoperated patients. Around 60 percent of operated patients got some benefit. The critics of psychosurgery ignored that. But their loss of social control made me feel less than good about this operation.

And as for the Freeman ice-pick operations. It was awful. Ugh. I got sick. I couldn't watch it. None of us could very easily. I saw it done once by Freeman at [Columbia] Physicians and Surgeons in New York and I had to walk out of the room. Walter Freeman was eccentric to say the least. I believe he probably had bipolar disorder, he was manic-depressive. He finally lost all his privileges at Georgetown and George Washington hospitals, although that was as far as people would go in stopping him. I don't have a very good answer to why he wasn't stopped, but I must say that the medical profession does a much better job in policing itself now than 30 years ago.

In 1961, Ballantine went to a meeting of the American Association of Neurological Surgeons, then known as the Harvey Cushing Society. One of his colleagues, Alan Fulkes, gave a paper on treatment of chronic pain with cingulotomy—or what they then called cingulumotomy—placing lesions, or cuts, in the cingulum.

BALLANTINE: He reported on sixteen cases with good results in over 60 percent. Four patients in that group had pain of unknown etiology. No one was even sure they had pain. Yet these four showed more improvement than any other. So I began to wonder if indeed they were operating for pain or for depression? Or a combination of both.

I went back and did a little reading of the literature and I learned that Sir Hugh Cairns at Oxford had been doing cingulectomies—that's removal of the whole front portions of both cingula—for psychiatric illness. He in turn had been stimulated to do this by John Fulton, a great physiologist at Yale University who was one of the pioneers of psychosurgery. Fulton's studies had suggested it might be enough to operate only on the cingulum and leave the frontal lobe alone, to get benefit in psychiatric patients.

He said this because in patients who had died from other causes but had done well following lobotomy, the cingulum had been interrupted in almost every case he could find. So he reasoned, avoid the antisocial aspects of lobotomy and just do the cingulum. Then a real red brick psychiatrist named Morris Flanagan, who had been an ivory tower guy before he went into private practice, opened a private sanatorium in Waltham [a suburb of Boston], and I sent several patients out there for treatment of serious depression. Later, I told him about a paper I'd heard the year before on the stereotactic version of Cairns's procedure. That was in 1962 now, and I told Flanagan it sounded reasonable. Cairns did it as an "open" operation, that is opening the skull to visualize the brain, but now there was the stereotactic version, which was much less damaging. In any event, Flanagan said okay he would be willing to see what kind of results he would get with this and that's how that procedure got started in Boston.

Ballantine recalls that people were very upset with him and others over this kind of work. But he never stopped operating. Even when, as president of the International Society for Psychiatric Surgery in 1979, he and other psychosurgeons were picketed at a society meeting. Along with Vernon Mark, Frank Ervin, and William Sweet, he was accused of wanting to use psychosurgery to control violent criminals, drug addicts, and other social undesirables.

BALLANTINE: People who are violent in a self-destructive way, suicidal because of psychotic depression or assaultive because of epilepsy, are certainly candidates. But what you're talking about, the way you put that, is a problem.

Partly, it's a question of semantics. What kind of violence are you talking about? If someone because of psychosis or brain damage tries to hurt himself or others, that type of violence is not a contraindication for surgery, as long as it is accompanied by clear-cut psychiatric symptomatology, leading toward a diagnosis of affective disorder.

But there is no sense in talking about people with character disorders alone, people who are just cruel to others. Mark and Ervin hurt the case for psychosurgery because of their ill-conceived statements about violence and the brain and surgery to treat it. They chose the time of the Detroit race riots to propose that a substantial proportion of violent behavior is caused by subtle or not-so-subtle abnormalities of the brain's limbic circuits and disease like epilepsy in the emotional part of the brain. Their timing was ill advised. But if you look at this from a purely scientific point of view, Mark and Ervin were probably correct in that among those rampaging mobs in Detroit they talked about, there were undoubtedly some mentally disturbed patients who could benefit from psychosurgery. Some people, of course, are just bad actors. They have a character disorder that has nothing to do with abnormalities in the brain or psychosis. No surgery can deal with that. It also seems true that most of the patients we operate on do not have an absolutely clear-cut diagnosis of one particular psychiatric disorder. They are very complicated psychiatric patients, and it's hard to sort out whether the dominant problem is anxiety, depression, or paranoia. They all can exist in one patient. We have one boy, the son of a physician, who is clearly schizophrenic, but with such overwhelming anxiety and fear that he was breaking windows and doing all sorts of bad things. Cingulotomy doesn't help schizophrenia, but we operated on him with the blessing of the psychiatrists. He is still schizophrenic, but he is not so violent or fearful. He's about 22 or 23 now and not functioning very well, but he's far less destructive.

Ballantine says the future of psychosurgery is light if not bright:

> Look at the way we treat psychiatric illness now without surgery. There's not a drug on the market without a side effect. I think the immediate future is refinement of technique so that we say for certain we have interrupted the cingulum completely.
>
> Many are looking forward to the elimination of all ablative procedures and toward a day when we can interrupt bad circuits by putting drugs *in* to parts of the limbic system that seem to be either stimulated or depressed. And that's an exciting field to contemplate. Then, of course, there is the possibility of some type of implantation. We have to go hand in hand with the neuroscientists to discover which areas and which neurotransmitters in what numbers are involved in particular psychiatric illnesses. But right now, for the time being, I would like to tell people that there is good evidence that this type of limbic system surgery can help six cases out of ten. If you have exhausted other forms of therapy and a psychiatrist agrees he has nothing else to offer and you are still disabled, you can think very seriously about surgery, because one thing we do know at least about cingulotomy is that it is safe, even if it is not always effective.

For Ballantine and those like him, most of today's psychosurgery should no longer be considered experimental in the broad sense of the term, but should instead be considered the treatment of choice among those patients for whom there is no other predictable, reasonable means of relief. Those who believe psychosurgery is too risky to ever be an option too easily forget that any treatment of any illness carries risk, and that the patient often defines risk far differently than those with no vested interest.

When scientists today use the word *experimental* to describe an innovative treatment, they mean the treatment's effectiveness, safety, and predictability carry some uncertainty; that they are not meant to be routine. The term does *not* mean the treatment is a wild guess without standards, or tough criteria, to meet; nor does it mean the same as "high risk." As medicolegal expert Michael Shapiro points out, "There's a difference scientifically and legally between high-risk procedures and experimental procedures." Heart transplants, for example, are considered high risk, but no longer experimental, and insurance companies in many states now pay for them because they are no longer unproven. In Britain and the U.S., psychosurgical procedures often are covered as well.

With operations for psychiatric illness, "experimental" also refers to the fact that science does not completely understand *how* or *why* the operations work. Nor do neurologists, psychiatrists, and surgeons always know which patients are never likely to benefit.

Some groups still use the experimental argument with great success, hiding their real agenda—to banish psychiatry and any form of mind therapy but their own version. L. Ron Hubbard's Dianetics program and the so-called church of Scientology are built on the premise that all "somatic" treatments of mental illness are evil and sinful. Hubbard was a science fiction writer who had psychiatric illnesses when he was young and was terrified by the prospect of ECT and psychosurgery. He invented Dianetics as an alternative to psychiatric treatment and later transmuted it into Scientology, to make it tax-exempt as a religion and end charges that he was practicing medicine without a license. Dianetics and Scientology sell and promote mechanical devices such as the "E Meter," which the program claims will cure or control psychiatric symptoms. (It's worth noting that no mainstream religion expressly forbids psychosurgery.)

By the broadest definition, psychosurgery remains experimental, particularly because its effects are permanent and irreversible.

However, the success of small lesions made in the brain to treat obsessive-compulsive disorder, panic and anxiety psychosis, aggressive behavior, and deep depression is arguably proven. As a treatment of "last resort" for a hard core of patients who've tried everything else, including drugs and electroconvulsive therapy, psychosurgery has a place as well. What's important to keep in mind, the experts say, is that in medical care, uncertainty comes with the territory. There is no such thing as a risk-free therapy and many medical and surgical treatments we take for granted are no more or less "experimental" than the most advanced forms of psychosurgery. Medical science is not exact, and progress depends on innovation and constant changes in hypotheses and protocols. No treatment has ever come to the health care marketplace with every question answered, every risk abated, and safety and effectiveness proven beyond a shadow of a doubt.

In his book on psychosurgery's dark history, *Great and Desperate Cures*, Elliot Valenstein writes, "It is much easier to criticize past mistakes than to identify in advance which therapeutic risks should be taken." There are not now, nor are there ever likely to be, "any scientific or ethical principles that will enable us to make the necessary predictions and decisions" about the value and use of innovative therapies. The more desperate the illness, moreover, the greater the willingness to take risks. "While the quality of the scientific rationale advanced to justify any innovative therapy must be considered, it cannot be the decisive factor," Valenstein notes. "Not only will knowledgeable people differ in their evaluation of any hypothesis, but, even more important, too many medical treatments have proven useful even though the scientific arguments used to justify them initially were later proven false."

For example, Valenstein estimates that 70 percent of psychiatrists consider ECT helpful for intractably depressed patients, even though the original rationale justifying its use has long since been discounted and despite the fact that no one can really explain its success. Aspirin and most of the drugs used to treat mental illness would also qualify as "experimental" in some respects. Aspirin is highly toxic, its effects diverse, and its use completely uncontrolled; psychoactive drugs are unpredictable, often abused, and dangerous for many. "If we were to reject treatments whose effects we did not understand, even aspirin would not have been acceptable during most of the period of its use," Valenstein says, and "despite the enormous amount of research on the biochemical action of psychoactive drugs, there is no agreed-upon explanation of how different drugs help anxious, depressed, manic, obsessed, and schizophrenic patients."

These medicines are used millions of times each day because they *work,* not because of "any compelling scientific rationale," he concludes. Much the same case can be made for psychosurgery's early use and the excitement it generated. In short—it worked, at least enough of the time to keep interest high. "In medicine, we have to be most influenced by the quality of the empirical evidence that a treatment does more good than harm," he says.

The few groups—primarily in Boston and London—doing the newer, safer psychosurgeries have consistently good outcomes, but the number of patients is small and the journals reluctant to publish a great deal about them. As a consequence, indications for psychosurgery remain highly controversial and narrowly circulated. Very few young surgeons even care to get involved, because there is no demand, and the cycle of ignorance, fear of backlash, inexperience, and political pressure keep patients from asking about it. In today's political and legal climate, doctors and hospitals also find it extremely difficult to do controlled, randomized trials of new procedures, especially for psychiatric disorders whose diagnosis is often subjective and vague. Psychological tests used to evaluate patients before and after treatment are "soft" at best, making "proof" of outcomes fragile.

What may draw psychosurgery back into the mainstream of medicine is progress in the broad area of brain science, rather than in the operating room. California psychiatrist Louis Jolyn West calls the kind of thing that Sol Snyder is doing at Hopkins with the cultivation of brain cells an example, as well as discoveries about the treatment of Parkinson's disease (PD) and other movement disorders that have links to the limbic system.

"Just consider the implications of the surgical interventions now under study for PD that were unthinkable not so long ago," says West. "Oftentimes the earliest symptom of PD is depression and who knows how much we'll learn about neurochemistry of depression at the molecular level with the help of Sol's work. That's the kind of thing that could lead to surgical treatment as a means of implanting medications or neurotransmitter supplements. That would make psychosurgery constructive, not destructive. Anyone who would try to foreclose the prospect of a surgical approach to an illness or disease of the brain that affects mood or behavior just isn't keeping up with science."

"If I had one message to send," says British psychiatrist Paul Bridges, "I would tell people that the kind of procedures we do here at Brook Hospital are safe and help a lot of people with extremely severe illnesses. I would tell people to take it seriously and that they can come here if they can't get it at home."

If modern psychosurgery mostly passes the "experimental" test with respect to treatment of last resort, what are we to make of those critics who claim that there is still serious danger that some doctors or governments may use psychosurgery for punishment or mind control experiments? The consensus is that the risk may be Lilliputian. But the rhetoric is so Brobdignagian that attention must be paid to the fear it generates. Once again, any danger must be viewed in relation to the benefit of some patients. The minds in question belong not to analytical jurists and ethicists, but to very sick people.

Some philosophers, ethicists, lawyers, and psychiatrists argue that even the techniques of psychotherapy used to help people with neuroses or to work through bad times in their lives are methods of controlling people, a way of getting someone (the patient) to do someone else's bidding (the therapist's). Intensive psychoanalysis, for example, can vastly influence values and attitudes and change people's lives forever, not always as they or their families might wish. Behavioral therapists, disciples of Ivan Pavlov and B. F. Skinner, are highly skilled at "extinguishing" behaviors, including phobias, anxieties, and inappropriate sexual activity ranging from homosexuality to pedophilia. They do this by reinforcing behaviors they want with rewards of one kind or another and by not reinforcing or by applying "punishments" to behaviors they don't want. "Aversive" therapies, which are very controversial, have applied small, measured, consistent doses of pain to stop even more harmful (in someone's opinion) behavior with great success. But the question is whether those techniques are or can be abused to satisfy a government, an institution, or an individual's desires to control ideas or behavior.

Broadly defined, behavioral modification can be said to cure mental disorder, protect the public, protect a person from himself or herself, or make a person easier to live with in institutions or outside. Regardless of the goal—profound or trivial—the issue is *who* decides if someone's behavior should be or can be controlled? Who gets "treated" or not? Who controls the means of treatment? A doctor, a psychotherapist, a hospital, a judge? Your mother, your spouse, the prison warden, the government?

Can these decisions safely stay in the hands of the "experts"?

Can a criminal refuse drugs to "tame" him even if he is a menace to other inmates or himself? Is he really a menace or are the guards merely irritated and looking for a way to ease their lives? What if his refusal means he is locked up in solitary confinement? Is that cruel and unusual punishment if he is mentally ill? Who, in this case, is controlling whom? Is Johnny required by the school to take drugs for his "hyperactivity" as the price of admission, even if his parents believe he is merely a normal, rambunctious boy? What of the private psychiatric hospital that collaborates with parents to commit a teenager who "misbehaves"?

The extreme view holds that coercion or the "aura" of coercion—the implied threat of retribution—is at play with all patients or prisoners who "accept" any form of psychiatric intervention.

What troubles these critics most, they say, is not that society has a legitimate reason to control the behavior of some people, but that those who "own" the means of control are not honest, that they have "hidden" agendas as well.

In a landmark article on the issue of mind control and psychosurgery, Willard Gaylin, M.D., told the story of a distinguished brain researcher (probably José Delgado) who was describing the potential use of remote-control electrode implants in the brain to control antisocial behavior as a humane alternative to imprisonment. Asked whether he would be willing to turn the control box over to the patient (who, presumably wanted to be a good guy), he quickly said no. Why not? "Because it's my box," he replied.

In the 1970s, no name was more prominent in the mind control debate than that of José M. R. Delgado of the Yale University School of Medicine. In a dazzling series of experiments on animals using electrical brain stimulation, he demonstrated how simple it is to overwhelm an animal's instincts and will. With his remote control implants, he stopped a bull on a rampaging charge in its tracks with a radio signal that stimulated a part of its brain. Monkeys could be stimulated to constant, intense pleasure. It was Delgado's philosophy and his vision of the future that fed many of the fears that exist today. As writer Maggie Scarf noted in the *New York Times* (November 15, 1970), Delgado envisioned a "psychocivilized society whose members would influence and alter their own mental functions to create a happier, less destructive and better balanced man." "The human race," Delgado told the *Times,*

> is at an evolutionary turning point. We're very close to having the power to construct our own mental functions through a knowledge of genetics ... and through a knowledge of the cerebral mechanisms which underlie our behavior.... Not only our cities are very badly planned; we as human beings are, too. The results in both cases are disastrous ... I don't think we're condemned by our natural fate to violence and self-destruction.

Delgado invented a machine, called a stimoceiver, that stimulated the brain and received brain-wave signals, sending signals on three channels and receiving EEG recordings on three. With the stimoceivers implanted in monkey brains, he could manipulate their anger, rage, hunger, thirst, pleasure, and pain. In a circuslike routine, he could make them repeatedly yawn then growl. He firmly believed that such devices could keep assaultive violent criminals safe enough to walk the streets, and in a book called *Physical Control of the Mind,* he wrote a dreamy defense of such experiments and activities:

> The possibility of scientific annihilation of personal identity, or even worse, its purposeful control, has sometimes been considered a future threat more awful than atomic holocaust. The prospect of any degree of physical control of the mind provokes a variety of objections: theological ... because it affects free will; moral ... because it affects individual responsibilities; ethical ... because it may block self-defense mechanisms; philosophical ... because it threatens personal identity.
>
> However,... it is not knowledge itself but its improper use which should be regulated. A knife is neither good nor bad, but it may be used by a surgeon or an assassin. Psychoanalysis, the use of drugs ... insulin or electroshock ... are all aimed at influencing the abnormal personality of the patient in order to change his undesirable mental characteristics.... Suppose that the onset of epileptics attacks could be recognized by the computer and avoided by [electrical] feedback: would that threaten identity? Or if you think of patients displaying assaultive behavior due to abnormalities in brain functioning: do we preserve their individual integrity by keeping them locked up in wards for the criminally insane?

In a final finger to his critics, Delgado said; "I suppose that to primitive man the idea of diverting the course of a river would have seemed irreligious."

The impact of such language was heavy then and remains so. Dramatists and novelists still borrow its content for their "horror" stories. One of the latest to do so is Caryl Rivers, who, in her book *Indecent Behaviors,* has literally lifted scenes out of Delgado's lab-

oratory and imagination, with characters that would make Sven-
gali resemble Casper Milquetoast.

To critics of psychosurgery, Delgado's work and continuing
efforts today to map the brain's behavior centers are evidence of
the dangers of psychosurgery and other forms of mind control.
Civil libertarians quake in their amendments and even less dog-
matic individuals have reason to feel a chill. Some people, they
say, *want* to control people to their own ends or society's. In a
series of books, lectures, essays, and debates, psychiatrist Thomas
Szasz argues the outside limits of this fear. Claiming that there is
no such thing as mental illness, he believes that every person's
own state of mind is what it is and any attempt to alter the mind or
brain is the penultimate assault on individual sanctity. In this context, fears of mind control persist and attention must be paid. But
that does not make the fears rational or reasonable. Notes British
psychiatrist Bridges, the idea that all somatic therapies—drugs,
surgery, electroshock—are dangerous is absurd. "There is a moun-
tain of evidence to the contrary. You cannot define mental illness
out of existence and you cannot subdue or avoid inappropriate or
bad treatments by suppressing all treatment." The solution to
abuse is not to forego innovation or research, but to keep practitioners reined and committed to human dignity.

George J. Annas and Leonard H. Glantz, lawyers who played
key roles in forming medical protection laws, argue that in the
end, a person's "only real protection ... depends on the conscience
and compassion of the investigator and his peers." The medical
profession's Hippocratic oath to "first do no harm" has historically
proven to be the best safeguard, leading doctors to withhold dangerous procedures even when they might help and to avoid
putting their skills in service to obnoxious political, experimental,
or punitive ends. Those physicians who have done so at the behest
of the Nazis during World War II, for example, are exceptions to
the long rule of self-discipline and self-policing in the medical
professions.

Today, the professional ethicists are joined by a strong consumer movement in which malpractice lawyers, Ralph Nader–style advocacy groups, government oversight, a more vigilant press, voluntary health organizations, and a better-educated public look out for abuses. Nevertheless, the experts acknowledge that new technologies and a bad history justify even more formal safeguards, and stringent regulations. Public sensibilities, argue Annas and Glantz, "will no longer allow ... the unregulated research of scientists who [claim dispensation from regulations because] of the special nature of the human brain." And today, there are institutional review boards in all hospitals, stricter regulation of surgical practices, and laws and regulations in some states that govern or ban certain kinds of procedures—from abortions to psychosurgery.

Ethical guidelines and regulations can never become absolute rule books. Rule breakers ignore them. But they can, writes Valenstein, "help to clarify issues and to sensitize physicians and others to questionable practices.... [But] knowledgeable physicians may disagree about treatment. Some risks have to be taken and some harm will inevitably ensue along with some benefit." He goes on to say,

> I am confident that formal regulation of surgical and other innovative therapies now uncontrolled will ultimately prove preferable to the current random regulation by malpractice suits, political action, and economic pressures. It is to be expected that any controls will be resisted, with the arguments that they will hamper progress and deprive desperate patients of help, and that randomized controlled studies are unethical in that they deprive some patients of the benefit of treatment. My own view is that the negative effect of reasonable regulation is exaggerated, especially when compared with the control of uncontrolled experimentation.

Current regulations and guidelines are not terribly useful to those looking for absolute answers; they do, however, offer some safeguards and clues as to how we might rationally debate the question: Whose mind is it?

Today, for all practical purposes, only the desperate at the end of their ropes can get a psychosurgical procedure. The criteria set down by review boards, individual surgeons, psychiatrists, and neurologists are vague and daunting. For instance, all patients must be chronological adults; children almost *never* qualify, not even teenagers. They must have chronic (very long-term) tension, anxiety, depression, obsessive-compulsive disease, assaultive behavior, or other profound psychiatric symptoms. *Chronic* can mean anywhere from 2 to 20 years or more. They must demonstrate a history before the sickness of having been a well-adjusted, employed, socially supported, sexually healthy person. The idea behind these criteria is that people who were unable to cope with life before they got sick are unlikely to do well with rehabilitation after surgery. In recent years, this standard has become somewhat more flexible and stretched to include people who may never "make it" on the "outside" but whose lives can be considerably improved. And they must have been nearly totally "disabled"— whatever that means—for at least several years.

Beyond these requirements, candidates for psychosurgery must demonstrate an almost complete lack of response to all other treatments, including drugs, ECT, "talk" therapies, and behavioral modification. How long the treatments had to be tried and under what circumstances (in a hospital) is up for grabs. Suicidal tendencies (usually translated as having made at least one unsuccessful attempt) are often the deciding factor to proceed. Candidates must, if they meet all of these requirements, get agreement to the procedure by various boards and ethical committees in hospitals where the operations are performed. The physicians who know the patient well are usually not considered qualified to make the judgment. Lastly, the record has to show that every conceivable attempt has been made to get informed consent even from individuals who have severely disabled social and intellectual capacities because of their illness, long years of institutionalization, or drug use.

In the face of such "guidelines," many psychiatrists and surgeons retreat into vague generalities of their own. Michael Jenike, the Harvard Medical School psychiatrist who has helped hundreds of patients with obsessive-compulsive disorder obtain cingulotomies, says: "When should we do it [psychosurgery]? Well, it's indicated if people don't respond to other things. It's obviously not the first thing you do. But the side effects are very minimal. If people are totally devastated by something, you use what you can to get them better. There's always someone who says you can't do this, you can't do that, you can't do shock therapy or psychosurgery. But if you have to take care of patients, you have to do what's likely to help them. And it will always stir up some people who will say it's a terrible thing."

That kind of verbal sidestepping should not be necessary, for there is substantive information on which to base clinical decisions. In 1978, an American Psychiatric Task Force on Psychosurgery sent a questionnaire to 1,450 American and Canadian neurosurgeons with a 78 percent response rate and learned that the annual number of psychosurgical operations in the United States was about 300 and the results were largely very good. In 1987, Ballantine at Massachusetts General Hospital reviewed his results on the latest 198 patients followed for up to 8.6 years, most of them with depression, manic-depressive psychosis, and other psychotic disease. He reported that 13 percent fully recovered, 23 percent needed medication but were functioning normally, 51 percent had varying degrees of psychiatric disability, 17 percent were only slightly improved, and 6 percent had gotten worse. As many as 9 percent died by suicide later. That's a track record that would be the envy of many surgical procedures, in or out of the brain.

The unique justification for psychosurgery, Bridges wrote in the *Journal of Neuropsychiatry and Clinical Neurosciences,* is based on a simple clinical decision: If the operation is not done, the patient is subjected to extreme suffering, which is untreatable. "It is quite unreasonable to plan to excessively restrict or to abolish psychosurgery without suggesting alternative therapy, especially since the operations now available are so effective and safe." He describes what he considers a reasonable nonsurgical effort for suicidal depression as one and preferably two courses of ECT that are ineffective, nonresponse to tricyclic antidepressants at increasingly higher doses of up to 300 to 400 milligrams daily for at least six weeks, then the addition of lithium for perhaps two months without success, then a final round of lithium augmenters. At the outside, perhaps six months to a year will pass before assessment for psychosurgery, provided there is a long-term history of disease.

In the tradition of the doctor as final arbiter, the issue of informed consent gathers unusual dimensions. For example, a patient may, after getting full information about the risks and benefits, choose an operation and still be denied it if the medical and regulatory establishments feel it's "too soon" to try such a treatment. Is the consent any more "informed" if it's accepted a year later? Or two or three or five? More fundamentally, can candidates for psychosurgery ever truly give informed consent, particularly if they are institutionalized and feel compelled to "go along" with whatever their caretakers hand out in order to avoid angering them? Can someone ever get psychosurgery without being able to give that kind of consent? Can family members give it for them?

Again, the experts overall seem to feel they can, although in today's "sue-the-bastard" environment, hospitals and doctors go to unbelievable lengths to protect themselves and their doctors from charges of violating a patient's rights or proceeding with treatment a patient hasn't understood and approved. Many experts, including former editor of the *New England Journal of Medicine* Franz Ingelfinger, have argued that it is probably impossible to get really informed consent from *any* hospital patients, much less a psychiatric or mentally damaged patient, because of the control doctors always have over patients in their care. The legal system's response has been to add layers of interpretation and red tape to informed consent definitions and procedures. In its least complicated form, this means that a doctor must tell the patient and be sure the patient or the patient's legal guardian fully understands every single risk as well as the benefits of the operation.

In more complicated situations, this process can take on the complexion of absurdity. Barney Clark, the Utah Mormon dentist who became the first man in history to have a totally artificial heart implanted, for example, signed a consent form that was more than 14 pages long but which in essence gave him the absolute right to terminate the experiment at any time, which in effect would end his life in a bizarre kind of suicide. It was reported after his death at a conference on bioethics held in Utah that on several occasions, Dr. Clark demanded that the machine be turned off. He'd had enough. In each case, his request was denied. The grounds? His doctors agreed that anyone who would ask for such a termination is by definition not of sound mind!

The major effect of informed consent procedures is to keep the numbers of candidates small and the seriousness of the operations highly visible. In the case of prisoners, the effect is to all but ban psychosurgery entirely. Mass murderer Edmund Kemper III, who killed his mother, grandparents, and seven others, tried unsuccessfully several times to get the surgery, and neurosurgeon M. Hunter Brown offered to perform it in an effort to rid him of his murderous paranoia. But a California county superior court said no, that Kemper would have to prove he was mentally ill before he could consent to have psychosurgery because the law in California says no prisoners can possibly give informed consent to such a procedure unless and until the procedure itself is proved safe and effective.

Baruch Brody, a professor of biomedical ethics and director of the Center for Ethics, Medicine, and Public Issues at the Baylor College of Medicine, has written that the process of informed consent by a competent adult requires as a first step the ability to get information from the environment and the people in it. From there, the patient must be able to remember the information, make a decision, give a reason for it, and show that he or she is using the relevant information to make the decision. Brody's conclusion is that "every judgment about competency is a judgment about the degree of competency rather than an all or nothing judgment." No one is so competent as to be totally objective about his or her own decision to have drastic treatment.

It may well be impossible to get informed consent when someone is floridly psychotic or demented. But if someone is depressed or has obsessive-compulsive disorder, experts say his or her thinking is usually intact. "These people are working, have families, often do fine on and off," says Harvard psychiatrist Jenike. "They are normal apart from their disorder. The ability to give informed consent and the symptoms of disease [appears] to live in different parts of the brain. To put it crudely, if you had a broken foot, that doesn't mean you can't use your arm to write out your consent to have it treated."

Definitions and requirements for informed consent vary from state to state. In some areas, the right to informed consent overrides every other right and often common sense. Internal review boards and multidisciplinary committees have sometimes added so many layers of safeguards and so many lawyers to invoke them that even *asking* for informed consent can be punitive. The outcomes of legal cases involving informed consent and psychosurgery are hardly reassuring—to patients, society, or the medical profession. As the *Kaimowitz* case demonstrated, asking for informed consent for psychosurgery might always carry with it an implied threat or an implied promise.

Lawyer Samuel Shuman says that laws and cases like *Kaimowitz* that appear to defend human rights might in fact curb them, because they absolutely exclude prisoners or involuntarily confined patients from any chance to benefit from experimental or risky treatments. Lawyer Robert A. Burt goes even further. "To blanketly declare that the mentally ill can never give informed consent to any treatment because the brain is the diseased organ in need of treatment in the first place is crazy," he said. "What that would really mean is that no person suffering from any diagnosed mental illness can consent to any treatment for mental illness. So you could never get treated and you're always mentally ill. So good-bye. That's ludicrous."

The British, at least cosmetically, have a better way. In the UK, the Mental Health Act set down strict rules for consenting to psychosurgery and established a commission made up of people who are neither close to the patients nor experts in the disease. Essentially, however, they can do no more than ratify or not ratify the decision of the psychiatrists. But the board at least gives the illusion that consent was obtained and no one's rights were violated. As one psychiatrist put it, "They all pretend to see the Emperor's clothes so they can get on with the business of treating with consent." That's a practical solution, but not very popular. Most doctors just muddle through on a case-by-case basis.

When all else fails, a guardian or "surrogate" may give consent. Alex Capron of the University of Southern California Center for Law and Ethics, and an authority on bioethics and the law, says American institutions have begun to define circumstances in which a family member or a "stranger surrogate" (court appointed) has legitimate interests and concern; and to define how much consideration that person can give to suffering, well-being, and quality of life as well as hope for a cure or return of function. The surrogate also is more likely to allow his subjective view of what *he* thinks the patient might want if he or she was able to make the decision.

"Obviously," says Capron, "we have to be somewhat skeptical about surrogates, especially family members, because of all the concern that surrogates might decide things for their own benefit. The sick person might be a burden on them, on their finances, or their emotional stability. The courts have to decide, especially if the operation is risky, whether the surrogate wants a shot at restoring quality of life or function or whether he just wants control and some peace." The problem, Capron concludes, is that "we've never resolved issues like this for general purposes, although I think we're a little bit better at thinking about them and debating them."

The general public, and some members of the medical and legal professions, seem far less adept at distinguishing between the target tissue of psychosurgery and the purpose of it. *They focus on the brain, but ignore the mind.* These folks—backed by some laws—argue for a ban on any operations on the brain without the presence of distinct disease or abnormal tissue. As we've seen, however, the lines between behavior and biology, chemistry and emotion, are increasingly blurred by new knowledge of the intimate connections among these. Moreover, the argument that ethical treatment never destroys healthy tissue is patently untrue. In treating cancer, for example, surgeons and medical doctors almost always remove some healthy tissue to prevent spread, or give drugs that poison or damage healthy tissue in order to preserve life or function of other tissues or organs. In some cases, women have breasts and wombs removed not because they are diseased but because they are at *risk* of disease.

In the brain, tissues may look normal and have no frank disease. But that does not mean they *function* normally. The signals transmitted between and among them may be sabotaged by abnormal amounts of chemicals or by bad "wiring" that no one has yet been able to unravel. "Psychosurgery is likely to remain an emotional issue," says British psychiatrist Desmond Kelly, "because it is difficult to understand why any operation on a brain that appears microscopically normal should benefit psychiatric patients." But, he adds, "what may appear microscopically normal, may not be *functioning* normally." Even the brains of epileptics, even where seizures arise, may appear absolutely normal to the pathologist.

The ethical and legal problems involved in operating on healthy tissue are important to consider, but as medicolegal expert Shapiro notes, you don't always have to go for a cure of disease to have a procedure be ethical, moral, legal, justifiable. "Sometimes, the justification is simply that we know people get better or behave better or feel better when we touch the brain here or there," says Shapiro. "In the case of some epilepsy, for instance, we say this person's problem is caused by a disease even though we don't know exactly what's going on. But that person has a right to be treated if there's a reasonable chance the treatment will make him better." He also points out that some medical and surgical procedures are considered ethical even when they are done in the absence of any illness at all. "It's nice that surgeons are doing ethical analysis," says Shapiro "but it is *not* the case that every time a physician does something with a drug or knife or anything else that he does so with the purpose of curing or controlling disease." When doctors give heavy doses of tranquilizers to the demented with Alzheimer's or the violent in prisons, are they treating "disease" or "behavior"? When they give doses of drugs that potentially cause serious side effects in order to prevent high cholesterol and heart attacks, is that "treating" nondiseased tissue?

Cosmetic surgery is an oft-cited case of treating nondiseased organs and tissues. Do we argue that someone's ugly nose is a "diseased" organ? Or her flat breasts? "In these cases," Shapiro says, "you're not really fixing a problem in Point A in the brain [where a person 'senses' ugliness about his nose], but you're doing something to point B [the nose] to prevent the problem from being played out in the mind. You are not directly treating the condition, but the symptoms." Some would argue the same goal for psychosurgery. At the very least, it appears—to some—no more unethical.

The use of amphetamines to make National Football League players more belligerent on the line of scrimmage, steroids to build muscle, and drugs like Rogaine to grow hair are other examples of "treating" or "operating" on healthy tissue. So is the use of human growth hormone to increase height. Although there are those whose very short stature is severely handicapping, growth hormone has also been taken by those who just want to be six feet instead of five feet, ten inches. "Being short, being bald, being flabby aren't diseases, but they do cause psychological distress, or what may be called psychiatric symptoms," Shapiro notes, and people's behavior and psyche change when they are treated. They're often happier.

Transsexual surgery to convert a biological male to a female is a case of treating biologically normal tissue that horrified many. For sheer invasiveness and permanence, it certainly matches psychosurgery. Many of these operations were performed in the 1960s and 1970s at the Johns Hopkins Hospital and in Sweden. In some cases, surgeons not only used hormones to build breasts and remove facial hair from biological males, but also removed fully functioning penises and created artificial vaginas. Psychiatrists involved with the experiments claimed that the purpose of the surgery was to treat a psychiatric disorder in which the victims are actually females trapped in a male body. Studies however suggest that those who underwent the surgery made no better psychological adjustment to their lives than those who didn't.

Americans have a broad tolerance for "treating" or dosing nondiseased parts of the body or brain or permitting unrestrained behavior as long as it makes people happy. The use of mind altering and addictive drugs comes to mind. "Right now," Shapiro said, "I want a cookie, but although I don't think I'm 'sick' because I feel vaguely unsatisfied that I can't have one, some people take that position." There is no black-and-white set of rules to guide the goals of treatments directed at behavior. "We need to make distinctions, to make judgments. But it's complicated."

The key question is whether benefits outweigh negatives in any treatment to any part of the body or mind. An ethical rule of thumb: Any treatment or activity that reduces autonomy and increases dependence should be considered carefully. But if the goal is truly therapy and there is informed consent from the patient or those *morally* responsible for him or her, then surgery or other therapies designed to modify temperament or personality are not unethical.

In the final analysis, people whose minds are at risk may have a right to get treatment as much as to reject it. Lawsuits have been won by patients who can show they did not get the latest, best, or most skilled treatment; but as a rule, patients do not have a right to a particular treatment, nor can doctors be forced to give a treatment. Moreover, a strong sense of "paternalism" exists among the medical and legal professions that embraces the notion that some people know what's best for us even if we don't like it. Ethicists, lawyers, and the courts have ruled that a physician is under no obligation to provide a particular technology or treatment just because it exists if in his or her opinion it is futile or harmful or against his or her conscience.

It *is* in society's interest to protect some people from themselves at times, and whenever doctors and patients must decide whether to do a procedure or not, paternalism comes into play.

Is the patient sick enough to warrant risky treatments? What would happen if we didn't do the treatment? Would the patient stay the same for a long time? Or deteriorate rapidly? What is the benefit compared to the risk? Is a 50-50 chance of some benefit enough? How about 70-30? Or 20-80 if it's the chance of a *lot* of benefit?

The preamble to Oregon's statute outlawing psychosurgery is a stunning display of paternalism:

> Whereas it is acknowledged that the human brain is the organ which gives man his unique qualities of thought and reason, personality and behavior, emotion and communication. And indeed is that unique structure importing to man his soul and ethical being; and whereas these things being so, the free and full use of the brain is the absolute and inalienable right of each individual, a prerequisite for making choices ... whereas it is the policy of the State of Oregon that deliberate and irreversible alteration of either the structure or function of the brain to bring about control of thoughts, emotional feelings, or behavior of a human being shall not be considered except in the most extraordinary of circumstances when such drastic procedures are proposed as a necessary court of last resort to provide a person in need of special treatment with human care. [It is the] intent of this ACT ... to provide the strictest possible control over the advocacy and practice of operations specifically aimed at permanently altering behavior.

Can paternalism go too far? Easily. Many think the Oregon law crossed the line, as do antiabortion laws, statutes like those involved in the *Cruzan* case (which kept a vegetating woman alive for years), and the denial of psychosurgery to a self-mutilating mental patient who blinded himself with a combination of cigarette burns and head banging (in that case, because drugs didn't help, his parents and doctors agreed to try psychosurgery. But someone in the Virginia attorney general's office objected and the hospital and Washington *Post* raised hell. After five years of struggle, the family gave up trying).

Access to care could, Shapiro says, be considered a fundamental right, but society has a legitimate interest in limiting the availability of procedures that are troublesome, dangerous, or unproven. Especially if they could become widespread. Somehow, our value system tolerates "extreme" activities that are limited in number and rejects them when they become too visible. That's especially true of activities that become symbolic, teaching a forceful lesson and taking on a life and history of their own.

Suicide and assisted euthanasia are examples of such "symbolic" activities. "We know that doctors routinely 'let' people die in hospitals, quietly and without publicity," says Shapiro. "We accept a few quiet occasions when a husband helps his suffering wife to die as long it doesn't get widely communicated and openly conflict with our collective values. We look the other way at a few modified lobotomies in a few isolated cases. The whole thing becomes different when people perceive that their values are offended." The bottom line is that institutions and laws can and do deny patients treatments society considers beyond the pale.

On the other hand, psychiatry "grew up" as a specialty because patients demanded treatment for mental illness and mainstream medical doctors and surgeons wanted no part of it. The history of medicine is filled with instances when the "consumers" of health care, by strong advocacy, political pressure, and financial incentives, drew the attention of medical science to certain diseases or disorders and the way they were treated. AIDS comes to mind. So does the use of less mutilating surgery to treat breast cancer. In the 1920s, William Halstead developed the "radical" mastectomy. It cured a lot of women and for decades surgeons resisted any effort to restrict their cuts, and any effort to even study alternatives to a procedure that left women deformed and in pain. The women's movement, helped along by a few courageous surgeons and cancer specialists willing to try alternatives, forced the National Institutes of Health and the medical community to develop serious studies of more limited operations, and today, most women can achieve the same benefits with far less mutilation.

If mental patients and their guardians and advocates want psychosurgery more available in the United States, they will have to demand it; to make their voices heard. "Surgeons," says psychiatrist West, "aren't standing in line to do these operations." But if people are firm in asking about their availability, more doctors and more hospitals will make them available.

The overwhelming consensus among the psychiatrists and surgeons interviewed for this book is that patients are entitled to wider access to psychosurgeries, but that the operations must still be seen as a last resort. Both major textbooks on the subject in Britain advise postponing psychosurgery for at least one year after all efforts fail with other means. Nevertheless, there is some weakening of the position among the few surgeons and psychiatrists who have long, successful experience with psychosurgery for selected patients. Says Britain's Bridges, who has supervised dozens of limbic leukotomies, leaving patients warehoused for long periods because they are not yet at the "end of their rope" is inhumane. "I've had patients who were at the end of their string from the start," he says. "And what's so magical about a year? Why not ten months or thirteen? It's nonsense." He accuses many doctors of relying on "last resort" thinking because they are ignorant or fearful of political consequences if they say or do otherwise.

Writing in the summer 1990 edition of the *Journal of Neuropsychiatry*, Bridges says, "the topic of psychosurgery for the majority of doctors and for many psychiatrists is still surrounded almost impenetrably by controversy and dissent, [supported] largely upon lack of up-to-date knowledge and to some extent even on misinformation." Psychosurgery, he lectured, "is nothing more or less than neurosurgery performed to treat certain psychiatric illnesses. The use of a special name gives the impression that something other than neurosurgery is involved. From there it is only a short step to the bizarre idea that psychosurgery, quite unlike neurosurgery, is used for political ends involving social control and for the subjugation of women, since more women than men have these operations."

Where does the fear of being wrong or unpopular trample on rights to prompt treatment? How long is long enough for some therapies not to work? Traditionally, innovative or extreme remedies always begin in worst, "last resort," cases so that ethically, doctors are on firm ground, doing no ultimate harm because the patient was never going to get better anyway and was probably going to die of or with the disease. But as time progresses, if the treatments are successful, doctors are expected to treat less and less serious cases to give the treatment and the patient the best possible chance of a good outcome. In the case of psychosurgery, most psychiatrists acknowledge that by the time the procedures are performed, behaviors linked to long-term drug therapy, incarceration, and abandonment make rehabilitation far less likely than if the surgery were done sooner rather than later.

Even in Britain, says Bridges, rehabilitation is difficult because treatment is

> likely to be carried out for those with chronic and very incapacitating illnesses.... There will have been a major loss of confidence, significant institutionalization is likely to have occurred, and social function will probably ... have been reduced for a long period. Another problem that occurs with over half our patients is strife within the family because of chronic or persistently recurrent affective disorders. Children find these illnesses impossible to understand and they tend to become antagonistic to the disabled parent. Marriages are threatened, and in the worst sort of case, the patient may recover following surgery but by then they have no family to return to and no home because there has been a divorce and the house sold.... Especially with older patients, they may have to stay in hospital [even if the surgery is successful].

Moreover, as people age with their mental illness, their physical deterioration makes the surgery less likely to be successful or uncomplicated. "They can't handle the post-op rehabilitation," says Bridges. "The demented stop caring and don't do as well even if you stop the depression. Waiting has deprived them, possibly, of years of better quality of life. Many psychiatrists believe psychosurgery would have *much* better results if it were done earlier in the course of illness."

Said one doctor, "I've had people kill themselves between referral and the time of their appointment for evaluation. If you have people who are so deteriorated that they've lost all their support systems, you won't get such good results. When we say last resort, it doesn't mean that we leave the case until absolutely the end of the rope or the last possible moment before a suicide occurs out of total despair."

In Britain and in the United States, younger adults are being operated on; in some cases, older teenagers. The big motivator for earlier surgery is suicidal depression. Even the most demanding review boards pay attention to suicide attempts. And a growing argument in favor of earlier surgery is that patients whose conditions resisted drugs and ECT respond to both after surgery and extend the operation's benefits.

Whose mind, then, is it to deal with, alter, or put at risk? Whose is it to protect? Experts, including Shapiro, believe the Supreme Court is unlikely to decide any issues with respect to rights or limitations of psychosurgery, who can consent to it, who cannot. Nor is the court likely to ban it outright.

The National Commission for the Protection of Human Subjects of Biomedical and Behavioral Research in 1977 defined psychosurgery as brain surgery on normal brain tissues or diseased brain tissue if the primary object of the surgery is to control, change, or affect any behavioral or emotional disturbance. Under this definition, any surgery with a dual goal—for example, relieving seizures as well as emotional abnormalities—is considered psychosurgery only if the main reason for doing it is to influence the behavior or emotional distress. The commission also said psychosurgery included implantation of electrodes; direct stimulation of brain tissue by ultrasound, laser beams, or electricity; and the direct application of substances in the brain, if the main purpose is to change or control behavior or emotions. It excluded shock treatment and surgery for Parkinson's disease and epilepsy and said nothing at all about pain relief as a form of psychosurgery. A later amendment said invasions of the brain that cut nerve pathways that carry pain signals were not psychosurgery unless they were done to relieve the emotional response to chronic pain without stopping the pain itself.

Nothing much has changed since then. Capron, the bioethicist and lawyer who was head of the commission and drafted those recommendations, says in the last ten years, the only direct legal response with respect to any of this has been the passage of isolated laws restricting ECT (in Berkeley, for one) and the courts eventually struck that down. Efforts in 1982 by him and others to have the secretary of what is now the Department of Health and Human Services amend its regulations to remove regulatory ambiguities and barriers to further ethical research on the mentally ill and disabled got nowhere. Therefore, regulations guiding federally sponsored research on human subjects stayed as vague and restrictive as ever.

All that we can expect in the near future from the business end of the current regulations is an "advisory" role to help guide internal review boards in all hospitals to ensure that "appropriate safeguards have been included to protect the rights and welfare of subjects." But no guidance is given as to what those safeguards should be. They are solely intended to limit risk and do not take into consideration other important factors such as consent of emotionally or mentally disturbed patients or of quality-of-life issues. Nor do they place limits on using these patients in research not directly related to their own illness, not likely to cure them, and not federally sponsored.

In the United States, especially, ethical and social debates related to medical rights and restrictions tend to deteriorate from broad issues to fractious, factional arguments over absolute "rights" and "wrongs." Witness the debate over abortion, birth control research, and fetal tissue research. As a nation, we seem unable to allow multiple approaches to problem solving; to consider the exceptional cases as worthy as the average; to be humane as well as politically, judicially, or technically "right."

To give every individual absolute control of his or her own mind and body is a formula for chaos. Laws, guidelines, and ethics guide and teach us how to live with one another. For those whose minds we cannot truly understand, however, we are long overdue to listen also to what lies outside the mainstream of our comfortable rules.

CHAPTER TEN

PROMISES TO KEEP

The trouble is not in science but in the uses men make of it. Doctor and layman alike must learn wisdom in their employment of science.

—WILDER PENFIELD, M.D., CANADIAN NEUROSURGEON
WHOSE 1935 PAPER ON THE FRONTAL LOBES INSPIRED EGAS
MONIZ TO PERFORM THE FIRST LOBOTOMY

Lobotomies are gone. No one should miss them. Worries about permanent assault on the mind and brain endure and the word *psychosurgery* still evokes outrage. Neuroscientists trust they will find ways to prevent or treat all mental illness without cuts or harmful drugs. But there are signs, nevertheless, that brain surgery to stop or control psychiatric disease is earning a second look and a legitimate place in health care. The editors of the *Journal of Neuropsychiatry,* for example, recently told readers to forget "psychosurgery" and substitute "neurosurgical and related interventions for psychiatric disorders," or NRI. "The new language won't sell any ties," quips former American Psychiatric Association president Melvin Sabshin, "but it could affect a few scalpels." Psychiatry, he said, remains "rueful" about the past "but should be open to any treatment." Other signs are as substantive as they are symbolic.

At the world-renowned Johns Hopkins Medical Institutions in Baltimore, chief of neurosurgery Donlin Long and chief of psychiatry Paul McHugh support preliminary plans to convene and host a small, international symposium of outstanding neurologists, neurosurgeons, psychiatrists, and basic scientists. The goal is to explore the status and the future of NRI, and there is talk of seeking a modest grant from the National Institutes of Health. Harvard neurosurgeon Tom Ballantine, and Britain's chief psychosurgical advocates Desmond Kelly, Paul Bridges, and Geoffrey Knight say the time is right for them to meet. They would make the trip.

"Maybe it's time to get our heads out of the sand," Long told me during a lengthy session in his office. "This attitude of neglect and denial has been of tremendous detriment to some patients. If the gross lobotomies of the past actually helped, and they did, think what we might do today with less destructive lesions, electrical stimulation, and drug implants." At the same time, Long acknowledges the "political risk" of exploring NRI and the difficulty an institution will face in recruiting surgeons and neuroscientists to the field. "It would take a strong place, but our young colleagues should be encouraged to look into it. This could be very important." Hopkins, he said, with its enormous strength in biological psychiatry, neuroscience, psychopharmacology, and neurophysiology, could take it on. "If not Hopkins, then who?" he said with a twinkle.

Warming to the idea, Long suggested that surgeons and psychiatrists could "cross-train" in neurophysiology, neurosurgery, and behavioral psychology. "Our best candidates," he said, "might come from those who've worked with Parkinson's disease and other movement disorders; those who already are looking at the links between brain anatomy and chemistry and brain control of mind and body in animals and humans." A blueprint for an NRI program at Hopkins or elsewhere, Long continued, would call for information on why and how drugs act on particular areas of the brain; the "neurocircuitry" of psychiatric disorders; experts on what goes on physiologically and dynamically in mental illness; and specialists with PET and MRI and innovative minds to develop better diagnostic and surgical tools and approaches.

Reversing the antipsychosurgery trend will require experience, team building, research, credible evaluation of results, and satisfied customers, and more. Imaging methods that go beyond MRI, which can only see small clusters of cells and nerve pathways in a "warped" curve, limiting the surgeon's ability to convert MR images into linear stereotactic dimensions. Animal models on which surgeons and neurologists can thoroughly test operations. Gene transfer experiments to manipulate the biochemistry of behavior. Cooperation with scientists in countries where there is higher demand for psychosurgery and fewer restrictions on experimentation. And procedures that can be reversed. "If we're going to move psychosurgery along," says neurosurgeon Haring Nauta, "we need something we can turn on and off, like remote electrical stimulation. A lesion, like a diamond, is forever, but not so an electrical current."

Leadership for a modern psychosurgical symposium, Long insists, should come from psychiatrists with a deep knowledge of neurochemistry and physiology. "But they'd need cooperative neurologists interested in cognitive behavior and surgeons willing to become experts on the limbic brain. You'd also need an institutional commitment to absolutely pristine science and the guts to tell the Peter Breggins of the world to stuff it," he added, referring to psychiatrist Breggin's lifelong battle to ban psychiatric surgery.

"From a political standpoint," Sabshin says of Long's interest and concerns, "it's true that if you stick your head up out of the trench, you may get shot down. But as anyone familiar with trench warfare knows, you can use mirrors to see out of the trench, defend yourself, and take proper aim at a target. It will take some courage, but there are safeguards that can work without inflicting deadly prohibitions. It's time to have that meeting and to think through related policies."

Along with the medical profession's new attitudes and plans, information for the general public is being offered—cautiously, tentatively, but also hopefully. In April 1990, the BBC released the documentary *The Last Resort* about psychosurgery at Brook General Hospital in London. The film marks the first time anyone connected with the psychosurgery program in the UK had "gone public." According to Bridges, the work grew out of a physician education film the same producer had done for him. "He was casting about for a new project, and because of the sensitive job that was done in the educational film, we decided to take a chance. Up to then, we had completely turned our backs on the media because of the sensationalism they applied to our work." The first 20 minutes of the film is a straightforward, stark depiction of a severely depressed woman and the disability experienced by her and her loving family. It makes the point over and over that psychosurgery is the only hope left to her and similar patients, and keeps expectations low.

"Everyone could see that by the time the surgery came, there was clearly no other choice," Bridges said. The response from the viewing public and critics was positive. The Knight Unit for Affective Disorders at Brook received some 90 letters from patients or patients' families within a few months. Bridges asked all 90 to bring referrals from their doctors and promised them a fair look. "If these all are suitable patients, that's a huge lot who wanted to know these operations are available to them," Bridges said. "And who knows how many did not write. I would guess at least a third of the 90 have not received treatment they should have and we'll put that right."

The BBC program and media interest it is generating are likely to spread the word farther in and out of the UK. The trickle of referrals from the United States and Europe had already increased in recent years. And the scientific media are getting the word out as well. For years, journals generally rejected articles on surgery for psychiatric or behavioral problems unless their content was couched in "politically acceptable" language. *Index Medicus* had very little labeled "psychosurgery" and relatively little overall on operations that mentioned modifications of mood and behavior as "side effects" or "secondary goals" of the surgical treatment. National and international meetings of psychiatrists, neurosurgeons, and neurologists, moreover, offered no papers, panels, speakers, or symposia on the subject in a frank and open way. Now that is changing.

Two years ago, the annual meeting of the American Psychiatric Association in Montreal, for instance, featured London's Kelly, a strong and longtime advocate of psychosurgery. "That invitation was something of a breakthrough," Kelly said. "People are willing to talk about it. Things are melting and there is a slow trend in the direction of growing awareness of the value of these operations."

A bigger breakthrough occurred in the summer of 1990, when the editors of a new journal, the *Journal of Neuropsychiatry and Clinical Neurosciences (JNCN),* offered a group of articles and an editorial exploring and supporting modern neurosurgery for psychiatric symptoms. Beyond suggesting new language to describe the operations, editors Stuart Yudofsky and Fred Ovsiew published reviews by Bridges (who also is senior lecturer in psychiatry at Guy's Hospital in London) and by neurosurgeons Robert Martuza, Ballantine, and Michael Jenike at Harvard.

Bridges's piece summarizes recent experience at the Geoffrey Knight Unit at Brook General Hospital in London, where, over the last ten years, up to 50 psychosurgeries have been done each year. He concludes that "the indications for psychosurgery are now clearer and the operations are carried out only when all other reasonable treatments ... have failed." And he proclaims that with the "refined and relatively safe procedures done in Britain, psychosurgery's "ethical uncertainties and controversies virtually have disappeared" under the Mental Health Act Commission review process. The Harvard and Massachusetts General Hospital team reported its success with stereotactic radiofrequency thermal cingulotomy for obsessive-compulsive disorder in the 20 percent of OCD patients resistant to other treatments and driven to suicidal depression.

"Each article," the editors of the *JNCN* said, "invites both the reader and our field to reconsider the pros and cons of the most controversial intervention for psychiatric illness. We wish to take this opportunity to advocate reconsideration of neurosurgically related treatments of psychiatric disorders and to propose the renaming of this rapidly advancing therapeutic realm." These are hardly timid words in a timid publication. The *JNCN*'s editorial board boasts many of neuroscience's superstars, including Floyd Bloom, Lewis Judd, Eric Kandel, Solomon Snyder, Joseph Coyle, Nancy Andreasen, Frederick Goodwin, and serving as chairman of the board and president of the publishing company, Melvin Sabshin.

Yudofsky and Ovsiew proposed in their editorial that the term *psychosurgery* "not only is an imprecise and outdated one, but very much like the label shock treatment [in that] it also evokes emotions that cloud, rather than clarify, therapeutic options for our patients." Modern NRI, they said, does not presume to operate on the psyche, the mind, but is

> more commonly ... directed toward treatment of disordered behaviors, drives, and affects than ... [toward] the treatment of what is more conventionally considered ... so-called mental dysfunctions. Admittedly, the boundaries ... often are blurred, such as in the case of obsessive-compulsive disorder. [But] more important, as with other antique labels—such as lunacy, idiocy, and insanity—that have been wisely discarded ... because of imprecise and stigmatizing usage in the common parlance, the term psychosurgery is burdened by unfortunate associations with punishment and other social or political misuses, and with overuse in realms where there were, in fact clinical applications.

Further noting that, historically, new ideas and technologies that once were harmful may "with ensuing advances become revolutionary contributions," they advanced their new term NRI in the hope it "opens therapeutic considerations to a broader range of treatments that would include ... transplantation of living tissues (e.g., adrenal and other tissue for Parkinson's), implantation of electrical devices, and the use of micro-osmotic pumps to deliver medications directly to the brain."

What triggered their proposals, the editors explained, are technological breakthroughs such as MRI and PET for mapping the brain and pinpointing target tissues that contribute to abnormalities, as well as better instrumentation for surgery, including lasers, electric and thermal devices of the kind used on Matthew, microscopic ceramic rods containing radioactive material, and medication pumps.

Reassuring readers that the bad old days are indeed worthy of burial, the editors said that "modern medicine now functions ... with overseeing bodies and committees able to review data, to establish and weigh risk-benefit rations, ensure informed consent ... and adjudicate the vast array of ethical considerations." In a final homily, the editors noted that in 1912 Sigmund Freud urgently advised colleagues to "model themselves on the surgeon, who puts aside his feelings, even his human sympathy, and concentrates his mental forces on the single aim of performing the operation as skillfully as possible." Freud's exhortation, they said, upset a lot of those who treat and work with the mentally ill. They added:

> We, who in this editorial are proposing the reconsideration of such "great and desperate cures" [as psychosurgery] expect controversy and indeed disapproval as we urge our colleagues to consider not only the attitude but also the technique of the surgeon in the treatment of psychiatric disorders. Freud understood the severity and the immediacy of the pain and disability of his patients, who suffered from severe psychiatric symptoms and disorders and the intense demands these disorders placed upon concerned clinicians. Even today, safe and effective treatments are not available for many patients and this makes neurosurgically related interventions worthy of attention. If medical professionals as well as the general public can overcome outdated attitudinal barriers, we believe this realm may, in the future, offer a treasure trove of therapeutic opportunities for our patients.

Coupled with changing attitudes about psychosurgery in particular is a sea of change in the way the public feels about psychiatry in general. For a while, it seemed that the psychiatric profession would never recover from the blows it took from psychosurgery's downfall, the dumping of the mentally ill out of hospitals into ill-prepared communities, the failure of therapy against epidemics of drug abuse, alcoholism, and family disintegration, the feminist movement's rejection of Freud, and the proliferation of "fringe" psychotherapies throughout the 1970s. I myself recall that in 1978, the year Martin Gross's book *The Psychological Society* and Thomas Szasz's *The Myth of Psychotherapy* were published, it was open season on psychiatry. Using psychiatrists and psychotherapy as the bull's eyes in social target shoots became the national pastime. Social historian Gross argued that America was headed toward that sublime psychological state in which everyone is either a patient or a therapist, and at the end of the 50-minute hours, the participants simply would change seats. The Western world, he said, had redefined every human characteristic from anger, sadness, and anxiety as no longer a normal reaction to life's stresses, but as mental illness in need of treatment. Szasz, long a burr under his profession's saddle, proclaimed Freud a fraud and psychotherapy a sophisticated combination of witchcraft and religion with no basis in the art or science of healing.

Whether or not psychiatry deserved such abuse, these criticisms at their peak demonstrated a broad spectrum public disaffection and distrust of psychiatry and its practitioners. But that same year, biological psychiatrists and their colleagues in neuroscience began to fight back, demanding of themselves and others rigorous attention to scientific principles, credible evaluation of their therapies, and in the halls of Congress, funds for new research. Therapists were exhorted to lay off the psychobabble and to resist stereotyping and categorizing patients and dehumanizing their treatments. Said Gross, "Far too often, with whatever good intentions, we want outcomes in patients that suit our stereotypes more than the patient's own aspirations. We need not stamp and stomp and squeeze on people, nor try to engineer their souls into some preconceived AMA [American Medical Association] or American Psychiatric Association approved ... soul." The profession, he said, "must begin to police itself to weed out cultism and greed."

The rehabilitation of the psychiatric and neurosurgical community is not complete, but its foundations of solid research, academic rigor in medical schools, and stricter regulation of treatments are improving. Progress is underway and has at least a few brilliant champions, among them Guy M. McKhann, director of the Krieger Mind-Brain Institute at Johns Hopkins University. After more than a decade as director of neurology at the Johns Hopkins Medical Institutions, McKhann put together a team of neuroscientists—including psychologists, neurologists, neurochemists, neuroanatomists, imaging specialists, computer programmers, and animal researchers—to investigate the links between mind and brain. The institute's goal: to understand the normal mind and brain and how it develops, as well as what goes wrong. An intrepid sailor—he has crossed the Atlantic in a small craft—McKhann is known for his candor and good old boy sense of humor (he long displayed a "no bullshit" symbol prominently on his desk). Says McKhann:

> Let's forget the term psychosurgery. It's loaded. Let's say that for a number of situations or neurological functions that are global—and most emotions fall in that category—surgeons have developed procedures that modify higher cognitive functions.
>
> You can put an electrode in a particular brain region and stimulate it, and a patient can stimulate himself or herself to modify pain. And we could say that patient is going from a state of feeling pain to no pain. But we could also say the patient is going from a state of feeling unhappy to happy. Get my meaning? We can mediate behavior through neurosurgical or other means, but calling it psychosurgery carries too much bad baggage.
>
> Memory is another model for this kind of analysis. And Alzheimer's disease. We have a fairly good idea about what specific systems are involved in short-term memory. But with long-term memory, we are beginning to see that the systems involved are really quite global, pretty damned diffuse. If you look at where in the brain long-term memories are stored, you've got a lot of different answers. So, if you have a mechanism by which you're putting a lesion in the brain or stimulating it, it's conceivable that there are multiple regions in the brain that you could stimulate to improve memory. You'd probably be able to activate the cerebral cortex in ways that are either going to allow faster recall of

stored information or increase retention, both of which are going to be translated into having better memory. People in this field are actively talking about how can one preserve a particular function like memory on the assumption that the cells that are involved with it might be dying, like in Alzheimer's. With transplants of nerve cells, or factors that preserve cells. Is this a surgical approach to modifying behavior? Damn right. But we're staying away from the old bugaboos. We're much better off projecting these procedures around specific functional systems, not something so vague as emotions.

McKhann acknowledges fads in medicine and the damage they do to the profession and patients:

We've seen this happen a number of times. When someone is bringing in a new procedure and it starts to catch on, there is this wave of enthusiasm that sweeps over every guy with a knife, and he'll do it if you'll let him. We started to see that even in the United States recently with the transplantation of cells for Parkinson's disease. And every jackass you can think of did a few. In fairness, a number of people really are interested in the problem of Parkinson's and learning something. But others are interested in getting their name in the paper or on radio, and then there are those who recognize this is a way to make a buck. People in my business don't like to talk about it, but that's exactly what happens. And it's exactly what happened with psychosurgery.

He goes on:

We have much better systems in place now for protecting individuals' rights. They're not perfect by a long shot, but there is a stronger feeling in medicine today that you must have data to justify what you do. The forces generating this are the failures of the past like lobotomies and procedures that have not stood the test of time. We're getting good at asking those questions. The artificial heart experience is a good model. Medicine set up a system to do ten or so operations that could possibly help patients with a problem that could not be solved with other means. This provided a model for learning. And the lesson we learned was to go back to the drawing board. But just because it didn't work doesn't mean it was wrong, only that it needed more work and more questions answered before going ahead. Abuses of any technology are possible. But people shouldn't make too much of some of the fears that are raised. There have been a few stories, for example, about the prospects of using aborted fetuses to "harvest" fetal brain cells for brain transplants. Now really. If you knew anything about biology, you'd know that would be a very impractical venture. You could presumably use skin [if you have the genetic and chemical switches that turn on particular functions in all cells]. We're probably also going to see the end of permanent lesions in favor of transient, positive effects using remote-controlled stimulation. And ways of preventing unwanted behavior or effects. For instance, I think there is increasing evidence that someone who gets addicted to cocaine has a lifelong addiction; it's never gonna go away, but the brain's chemistry has been transformed. So the problem is to try to modify the behavior (taking the drug, getting the high) by changing what cocaine has done to the brain. The brain works in systems. And we now have to get back to the systems approach to tell us how the brain works. A lot of people recognize that now. At last.

Strident critics of psychosurgery will find even McKhann's scholarly, if sometimes intemperate, view of his science still terrifying "proof" that damaging the brain for any purpose is unthinkable.

Yet scientists will always do what they can do, which is another way of saying they can be counted on to take cunning advantage of tools at hand. With that leap of creative utility, the impossible or impermissible has a way of becoming feasible. Forty years ago, medical students were taught they could *never* operate on the heart. Today on the cocktail circuit, heart transplants are old news, and the talk is about tissue transplants for the brain. *In vitro* fertilization and surrogate pregnancies were outside the ethical pale less than a generation ago and today are ventures for entrepreneurs. Twenty years ago, gene therapy could be found—in the pages of science fiction. Doctors at the National Institutes of Health are now doing it. If there is a Murphy's Law of science, converting the unthinkable to household words is it.

And no where is it more certainly revealed than among those who study and treat the mind and brain. After centuries of culling all they could about the brain with the naked eye and intuition, scientists jumped on every new discovery in imaging, molecular biology, chemistry, and genetics to track down the nature and activity of what the brilliant Spanish neuroanatomist Santiago Ramon y Cajal almost a century ago labeled the "explored continents and unknown stretches" of the brain.

Today, Cajal's scientific descendents know the locations and functions of many of the 10,000 million neurons that lay embedded in what one writer has called the "three-pound universe." They know how many of these nerve cells—directed by dozens of chemical switches—operate the senses, store information, and direct motion and emotion. They've mapped some of the dense network of interlocking connections that carry millions of message-filled electrical signals through the brain and spinal cord. People who keep tabs on this sort of thing say that the publication rate among neurosciences is many times that of any other specialty in the life sciences and shows no sign of slacking off.

Inevitably, there were those who absorbed the new knowledge against the backdrop of old experience. One result is that the promise psychosurgery held out to its pioneers has in part held up, regardless of its subversion by overambitious practitioners. With the comfort and safety of passing decades, psychosurgery can be seen not as an abnormal blip on the scientific radar but as a somewhat expected curve on the road to knowledge.

In a 1988 essay on lobotomies in honor of John Fulton, whose experiments on the chimps Becky and Lucy uncovered the frontal lobes as part of our emotional circuitry, Jack D. Pressman explained, "As in the case of other popular treatments whose initial therapeutic esteem eventually soured, psychosurgery's sharp reversal in clinical fortune poses the difficult question: Why would reasonable, well-meaning physicians and scientists at first value a procedure so highly only to abandon it later as obviously meritless? It's neither enough nor accurate to say they 'came to their senses.'... At issue is the nature of medical progress."

The nature of that beast, Pressman went on, is that most medical innovations are initially tried *not* because they are first proven to be sound and effective; on the contrary, most "crash" and "appropriately find only oblivion," even if they start out being "sound," while others "seemingly unlikely in fact find their way into clinical practice and for a time are judged to be *bona fide* medical boons. To assume that when physicians consider a new treatment they somehow are guided by a special insight into its true clinical value—a value not yet determined—is to impose an unwarranted, although reassuring, teleology."

For those who investigate and try to order the mind—the very instrument we call on to bring order to our inquiries—the task is formidable and full of hairpin curves. Yet at worst, the "failed" therapy of psychosurgery holds value in revealing to us principles that lead to standard, successful medical therapies, the most potent of which is serendipity—accident that favors the prepared mind—followed closely by compassion and the guts to challenge the conventional wisdom.

Lobotomies and all of early psychosurgery were experiments that failed. But experiments are a scientist's way of asking questions. To achieve the new promise of psychosurgery without the abuses that wrecked the old, the questions—and their answers—must be smarter, better regulated, and carefully watched.

Most of us go through life never having to unbundle our biological and emotional parts. We move seamlessly between thoughts and feelings and movements. And although we may know intellectually that every single act—every twitch of the nose, every tear, orgasm, angry rage, and test answer—flows from neurons in our brain, we remain unaware of its power, taking for granted that our "wiring" is in place. For the mentally ill, the seams have come apart. Mind-brain scientists, including neurosurgeons, *must* search for the knowledge to help the mentally ill; and for the rest of us, to push knowledge of ourselves to new horizons.

GLOSSARY

WORDS AND TERMS ASSOCIATED WITH PSYCHOSURGERY

Affect: An emotional state of being, or mood. Affective disorders refer to such psychiatric illness as mania (inappropriate euphoria) and depression.

Amygdala: Two brain structures located in the temporal lobes that contain incoming and outgoing fibers that relay and regulate aggression and other intense emotions. They are connected to the hypothalamus directly by the septum pellucidum, which is concerned with pleasure reactions.

Axon: The part of the neuron, or nerve cell, that sends or carries messages from the body of the cell to its "tail," where they can be sent across "synapses," or gaps, to other neurons. The cell bodies reside in the cortex, caudate, thalamus, and other structures under the cortex.

Basal ganglia: Also called "striatum," these tissues are critical to the control and regulation of motion, sensation, and feelings. They contain many dopamine receptors.

Cerebellum: The central structure at the base of the brain that joins the main part of the brain and the brain stem, and is responsible for regulating and monitoring movement of the body, balance, and coordination.

Cerebral cortex: A thin, gray, quilted or wrinkled layer of nerve tissue that entirely covers the two halves or hemispheres of the brain. Often called the "gray matter," it is called cerebral because it is on top of the cerebrum, and cortex because it is the outer covering. The cerebral cortex is the brain's main information-processing tissue, made up of billions of cells held together with a gluelike group of cells called glia. The cerebral cortex sorts, collects, organizes, and sends all information to other parts of the brain and body, which people then recognize as sight, sound, feelings, and memories. In humans, this part of the brain is the most highly developed and is responsible for our higher intellectual functions.

Cerebrum: The dense layer of nerve fibers covered by the cerebral cortex and also known as the white matter.

Cingulotomy: Psychosurgery that involves cutting or severing tissues in the cingulate gyrus. It is the most frequent form of psychosurgery performed today.

Cingulum, cingulate gyrus, and cingulum cortex: Tissues that form the upper portion of the limbic system. The cingulate gyrus is an arc-shaped groove running along the lower side of gray matter of the cortex.

Corpus callosum: A C-shaped band of white nerve fibers that connects the left and right cerebral hemispheres.

CT scan: Computed tomography scan once known as CAT, or computerized axial tomographic scan. The technology uses computers to convert X rays of the brain into detailed pictures of separate brain structures. X rays can only highlight bone.

ECT: Electroconvulsive therapy, or "shock" therapy, this treatment sends measured electrical current through the temples to create a brain seizure. For unknown reasons, the treatment, which is done under anesthesia and is not painful to the patient, relieves profound depression.

Forebrain: One of the major functional and anatomical parts of the brain. The forebrain is made up of the cerebral hemispheres, the left and right thalamus, the hypothalamus, and the limbic system.

Fornix: A bundle of nerves leading from the hippocampus.

Hippocampus: Tissue in the lower arc of the limbic system involved with short-term memory, learning, and emotion.

Hypothalamus: Located under the thalamus at the base of the brain, it receives input from most other parts of the brain and regulates many body activities as well as the pituitary gland. This gland, also called the master gland, activates and produces many regulating hormones. Along with the pituitary, the hypothalamus is one of the major routes carrying signals of psychological stress—good and bad—to heart, lungs, bladder, and other internal organs.

Limbic system: Also called the "emotional" brain, this system is composed of the cingulate gyrus, septal region, fornix, mammillary bodies, and other structures that are rich in dopamine.

MRI: Magnetic resonance imaging was formerly known as NMR, or nuclear magnetic resonance. Using powerful magnets to line up magnet-sensitive molecules in the body's tissues, MRI uses computers to interpret the various concentrations of those molecules to give clear pictures of the brain and other parts of the body. Its advantage over CT scans is that is does not use any radioactive materials.

Neuroscience: Collectively, this refers to a group of scientific and medical disciplines devoted to the brain and how it works. Among the disciplines are neuroanatomy, the study of brain structure; neurochemistry, the study of neurotransmitters; neuropharmacology, the action of drugs on the brain; and neuropsychology, attempts to "map" or locate functions of the mind—thinking, feelings, motivation—in the brain. Many definitions also include psychiatry, neurology, and neurosurgery, the practice of medicine related to disease and abnormalities in the brain.

Neurotransmitter: A chemical "messenger" used by neurons to activate other messages or signals that control brain function. The better-known neurotransmitters include dopamine, norepinephrine, serotonin, acetylcholine, and GABA (γ–aminobutyric acid).

PET scan: Positron emission tomography is a brain scan made by using short-acting radioactive materials that emit positrons, which are picked up and measured by sensors and translated by computer into pictures of the brain. But unlike MRI and CT scans, PET highlights how the brain uses the substances injected for the scan, and thus permits doctors to study function as well as form.

Prefrontal leukotomy: Psychosurgery that involves cutting white matter tissue, also known as prefrontal lobotomy.

Temporal lobe: The side lobe of each major half, or hemisphere, of the brain, located at or near the temple above and around the bones that encase the inner ear. The temporal lobes are below the frontal lobes and in front of the occipital lobe, which rests above the cerebellum.

Thalamus: Located deep in the forebrain, the thalamus relays and receives messages from other areas of the brain.

Appendix A: Rehabilitation After the Psychosurgical Operation of Stereotactic Subcaudate Tractotomy in the United Kingdom

Rehabilitation is of particular importance after psychosurgery because this treatment is likely to be carried out for those with chronic and very incapacitating illnesses. This means that there will have been a major loss of confidence, significant institutionalization is likely to have occurred, and social function will probably have been seriously reduced for a long period. Another problem that occurs with over half our patients is strife within the family because of chronic or persistently recurrent affective disorders. Children find these illnesses impossible to understand and they tend to become antagonistic to the disabled parent. Marriages are threatened and, in the worst sort of case, the patient may recover following surgery but by then they have no family to return to and no home because there has been a divorce and the house sold, perhaps. This scenario makes rehabilitation very difficult and, again in the worst circumstances, we have known the operation to succeed in stopping depression but rehabilitation did not succeed for social reasons such as those described. Especially with older patients, they may have to stay in hospital nonetheless. (The treatment was a success but rehabilitation failed.)

However, there are special aspects to rehabilitation after psychosurgery and these stem from two opposing factors. Firstly, as we make clear to all patients, the response to the operation is usually slow. The symptoms tend to fade gradually over a period of weeks or months. The opposing observation is that patients have marked "cognitive" lag after psychosurgery. Even soon afterward, other patients and the staff can very often observe less retardation and more social communication but the patient can be totally unaware of this improvement.

Thus, rehabilitation has to be a slow process because recovery is slow but, nonetheless, the patient's assessment of their own recovery cannot be relied upon because of impaired insight and it is likely to be unnecessarily pessimistic. In essence, rehabilitation must be gradual but usually not as gradual as assessed by the patient's complaints.

The cognitive lag can be very difficult to counter. The best way to assess it is to encourage the patient, at an appropriate time after the operation, to carry out an activity that has not been possible for a long time. This might be something as simple as leaving the ward. The patient will protest that it is not possible, but with a great deal of support and encouragement the patient finally attempts and succeeds. The patient is congratulated at doing something new but the reply almost invariably is that well yes, they managed it but still they feel no better. This sort of conversation is quite characteristic and, for example, we have pointed out to a patient that he has been on a bus for a short journey for the first time in many years but this does not seem to produce rejoicing. The reply is yes, but it was a lot of effort, he feels no better, and would not wish to try again.

We once operated on a lady in her late 30s and she returned home to a rather isolated part of the country where regular psychiatric support seemed difficult to set up. In any case, one of her problems was getting out of the house. When we reviewed her one year after psychosurgery she remained almost completely housebound although anxiety and depression were very much improved. This turned out to be simply a failure with rehabilitation because regular professional help was not easily available to her. We admitted her to our Unit and we, in effect, trained the husband to carry out rehabilitation by taking the patient out for short distances at first and then for longer distances, then taking her to shops and later encouraging her to go into shops by herself. We did not see the patient for another year although the husband was encouraged to telephone us to report progress, which he did. Two years after the operation the patient was functioning almost normally.

It is these general principles that are important rather than the availability of rehabilitation facilities. The process involves increasing socialization, increasing independence, increasing confidence and help with the return of social skills.

MEDICATION

It was our policy at one time for medication to be stopped just before or soon after the operation, and it was only resumed if necessary. Now that it is entirely clear that most patients do not recover quickly, we now usually continue the medication postoperatively that the patient was admitted on. It should be possible to progressively reduce the tablets as increasing activity occurs.

Appendix B: Information for Patients: The Psychosurgical Operation of Stereotactic Subcaudate Tractotomy

This is an operation that is sometimes performed to help patients suffering from psychiatric illnesses who do not respond adequately to other treatments, such as drug therapy and electrical treatment (ECT). It is mainly available for patients who are suffering from severe depressive illnesses but under certain circumstances it may be helpful for chronic anxiety or obsessional states.

ASSESSMENT FOR THE OPERATION

Patients who wish to be considered for the operation are assessed at the Geoffrey Knight Unit by a team including a consultant neurosurgeon and a consultant psychiatrist. Relatives are invited to attend the assessment and to discuss their view of the problems with the Unit's social worker as well as with the doctors. The initial assessment is usually made on an outpatient basis, lasting about one hour on a Thursday afternoon. Sometimes patients are admitted for about two weeks for a more detailed assessment.

At the first consultation the operation of stereotactic tractotomy may be suggested or the doctors may recommend another form of treatment such as different medication or a further course of ECT, which should be tried before considering an operation. Less commonly, a decision may not be possible without results of further special tests such as a head scan.

PROCEDURE IF AN OPERATION IS RECOMMENDED

If the consultant neurosurgeon and psychiatrist agree that it is appropriate to offer an operation, and the patient wishes to have surgery, then the case is referred to the Mental Health Act Commission (this is a body set up by Parliament to protect patients' rights), who appoint three Commissioners to visit the patient. By law, a patient can have this operation only if the Commissioners are satisfied that:

> 1) it is a suitable treatment for his condition and
> 2) the patient wants this treatment.

In order to decide this they usually interview the patient at home or in his local hospital.

ADMISSION FOR STEREOTACTIC TRACTOTOMY

When the Mental Health Act Commissioners agree that an operation can be performed, each patient is allocated an operation date, and is admitted to hospital ten days before this for various tests including blood tests, X rays, and scans.

THE OPERATION
Procedure

The operation is performed under general anesthetic; it usually starts at 8.30 a.m. and lasts one and a half to two hours. The hair on the head is not removed. Patients are normally awake by lunchtime and can begin to eat and drink by the evening of the day of operation. It is only necessary to stay in bed for a short time after the operation and most patients are up and about on the second day after the operation.

Patients often complain of headache immediately after surgery, but this usually settles in a day or so.

TECHNIQUE

The operation aims to sever nerve pathways in the brain believed to be involved in psychiatric illnesses. It uses a safe, accurate technique and we have now carried out more than 1,000 operations. The horizontal incisions are made in the skin creases on each side of the forehead a few centimeters above each eyebrow. Then a small hole in the bone is made on each side. Tiny rods (7 mm X 1 mm) of a radioactive material called YTTRIUM are inserted using a fine hollow needle and X-ray pictures are taken to ensure accurate placement. The radioactivity lasts for only 1–2 days and only affects the tissue within 1–2 millimeters of each rod. The incisions are closed with stitches that remain in place for two days. The scars are obvious at first, but within a few weeks they tend to fade. In most cases they are hardly visible as they are usually hidden in a normal skin crease and therefore leave virtually no sign of the operation.

Postoperative procedure

Patients remain on the ward for at least two weeks after the operation and usually return to their local hospital for rehabilitation. Improvement is usually gradual over several months. As progress occurs the patient is encouraged to return to normal activities and to spend increasing periods of time at home. Medication is usually continued for several months at least.

Patients are asked to return to the Brook for an assessment of their progress at six months and one year after the operation.

RISKS OF OPERATION

The commonest adverse effect following this operation is an epileptic fit, which we know to have occurred in about 2% of patients (an epileptic fit occurs in 0.5% to 1% of the normal population). Most of these patients will suffer only one such fit but where more than one has occurred this tendency may be controlled with medication.

Any operation on the brain carries a small risk of very serious complications such as hemorrhage to the brain or infection but these are, fortunately, rare and in the case of this operation only one patient in over 1,000 has had a major hemorrhage. Of course such serious though remote risks have to be balanced against the possible benefits. It is our belief that the patient must be the one to make this particular decision.

OUTCOME AFTER STEREOTACTIC TRACTOTOMY

This operation produces full or almost complete recovery in about 50% of those patients who are selected by this Unit and accept our offer of operation. A further 20–30% of patients experience some relief from symptoms but do not recover completely. However, with these patients medication that was not producing benefit before the operation may be more effective afterward. Another 20–30% of patients do not change as a result of the operation. However, there is NO evidence that stereotactic tractotomy causes a worsening of symptoms.

While patients who have an illness that is likely to respond to the operation are selected it is not yet possible to predict which of these patients will benefit most. Thus, stereotactic tractotomy must be undertaken in the knowledge that it may not result in recovery.

Appendix C: Mental Health Act 1983, United Kingdom

Part IV
Consent to Treatment

56.—(1) This Part of this Act applies to any patient liable to be detained under this Act except—

(a) a patient who is liable to be detained by virtue of an emergency application and in respect of whom the second medical recommendation referred to in section 4(4)(a) above has not been given and received;

(b) a patient who is liable to be detained by virtue of section 5(2) or (4) or 35 above or section 135 or 136 below or by virtue of a direction under section 37(4) above; and

(c) a patient who has been conditionally discharged under section 42(2) above or section 73 or 74 below and has not been recalled to hospital.

(2) Section 57 and, so far as relevant to that section, sections 59, 60 and 62 below, apply also to any patient who is not liable to be detained under this Act.

57.—(1) This section applies to the following forms of medical treatment for mental disorder—

(a) any surgical operation for destroying brain tissue or for destroying the functioning of brain tissue; and

(b) such other forms of treatment as may be specified for the purposes of this section by regulations made by the Secretary of State.

(2) Subject to section 62 below, a patient shall not be given any form of treatment to which this section applies unless he has consented to it and—

(*a*) a registered medical practitioner appointed for the purposes of this Part of this Act by the Secretary of State (not being the responsible medical officer) and two other persons appointed for the purposes of this paragraph by the Secretary of State (not being registered medical practitioners) have certified in writing that the patient is capable of understanding the nature, purpose and likely effects of the treatment in question and has consented to it; and

(*b*) the registered medical practitioner referred to in paragraph (*a*) above has certified in writing that, having regard to the likelihood of the treatment alleviating or preventing a deterioration of the patient's condition, the treatment should be given.

(3) Before giving a certificate under subsection (2)(*b*) above the registered medical practitioner concerned shall consult two other persons who have been professionally concerned with the patient's medical treatment, and of those persons one shall be a nurse and the other shall be neither a nurse nor a registered medical practitioner.

(4) Before making any regulations for the purpose of this section the Secretary of State shall consult such bodies as appear to him to be concerned.

Selected Bibliography

Abrams, Richard. *Electroconvulsive Therapy*. London: Oxford University Press, 1988.

Alexander, F. G., and Selesnick, S. T. *The History of Psychiatry: An Evaluation of Psychiatric Thought and Practice from Prehistoric Times to the Present*. New York: Harper & Row, 1966.

Andreason, Nancy C. *The Broken Brain, The Biological Revolution in Psychiatry*. New York: Harper & Row, 1984.

Andrews, Lori B. "Legal Considerations in Neurotransplants," presented at the annual meeting of the American Association for the Advancement of Science, New Orleans, LA, Feb. 20, 1990.

Andy, Orlando. "Thalamotomy for Hyperresponsive Syndrome." In *Psychosurgery*, E. Hitchcock et al. (eds.), Springfield, IL: Charles C. Thomas, 1972.

Andy, Orlando. "Neurosurgical Treatment of Abnormal Behavior." *American Journal of Medical Science*, vol. 132, 1966.

Annas, George, and Glantz, Leonard. "Psychosurgery and the Law's Response." *Boston University Law Review*, 1974.

Arnold, William. *Shadowland*. New York: McGraw-Hill, 1978.

Ballantine, H. T., "Neurosurgery for Behavior Disorders." In *Neurosurgery*, Wilkins R. H., and Rengachary, Setti (eds.) New York. McGraw-Hill Book Company, 1985.

Ballantine, H. T., et al. "Stereotaxic Anterior Cingulotomy for Neuropsychiatric Illness and Intractable Pain." *Journal of Neurosurgery*, vol. 26, 1967.

Ballantine, H. T., et al. "Treatment of Psychiatric Illness by Stereotactic Cingulotomy." *Biological Psychiatry* 22:807–819, 1987.

Barhol, H. S. "1000 Prefrontal Lobotomies—A Five to Ten Year Follow-Up Study." *Psychiatric Quarterly* 32:653–678, 1958.

Bartlett, J., Bridges, P. K., and Kelly, D. "Contemporary Indications for Psychosurgery." *British Journal of Psychiatry*, vol. 138, 1981.

Barraclough, B. M., et al. "Use of Neurosurgery for Psychological Disorders in British Isles during 1974–76." *British Medical Journal*, vol. 2, 1978.

Barth, J., et al. "The Effects of Prefrontal Leukotomy: Neuropsychological Findings in Long-Term Chronic Psychiatric Patients." *The International Journal of Clinical Neuropsychology*, vol. VI, 1984.

Benson, D. F., and Stuss, D. T. "Motor Abilities after Frontal Leukotomy." *Neurology*, vol. 32, 1982.

Bernstein, I., Callahan, W., et al. "Lobotomy in Private Practice." *Archives of General Psychiatry*, vol. 32, 1975.

Black, Donald. "Psychosurgery." *Southern Medical Journal*, vol. 75, 1982.

Breggin, P. "An independent follow-up of a person operated upon for violence and epilepsy by Drs. Vernon Mark, Frank Ervin, and William Sweet of the Neuroresearch Foundation of Boston." *Rough Times*, vol. 3, 1973.

Breggin, Peter. "The Politics of Psychosurgery." *Proceedings of the Fourth International Congress of Social Psychiatry*, 1972.

Breggin, Peter. "Therapy as Applied Utopian Politics." *Journal of Mental Health Society*, 1974.

Breggin, Peter. "The Return of Lobotomy and Psychosurgery." *Congressional Record*, Feb. 24, 1972.

Breggin, P. R. "Lobotomies; Alert, Letter to the Editor." *American Journal of Psychiatry*, vol. 129, 1972.

Bridges, P. "Psychosurgery Revisited." *Journal of Neuropsychiatry*, vol. 2, 1990.

Bridges, P. K., et al. "The Work of a Psychosurgical Unit." *Journal of Postgraduate Medicine*, 1983.

Bridges, Paul. *Psychosurgery Update*, 1984.

Bridges, P. K., and Bartlett, J. R. "Psychosurgery: Yesterday and Today." *British Journal of Psychiatry*, vol. 131, 1977.

Brody, Baruch. *Life and Death and Decision Making.* New York: Oxford University Press, 1988.

Brownfeld, Allan C. "Psychosurgery: Mental Progress or Medical Nightmare?" *Private Practice*, June 1973.

Burt, Robert A. "Why We Should Keep Prisoners from the Doctors. Reflections on the Detroit Psychosurgery Case." *Hastings Center Report* 5(1):25–34, 1975.

Cappabianca, P., et al. "Surgical Stereotactic Treatment for Gilles de la Tourette's Syndrome." *Acta Neurologica*, 1987.

Chorover, S. L. "The Pacification of the Brain: From Phrenology to Psychosurgery." In Morley T. P. (ed.), *Current Controversies in Neurosurgery.* Philadelphia: W.B. Saunders, 1976.

Consensus Conference Report. Surgery for Epilepsy, National Institute of Neurological Disorders and Stroke. Bethesda, MD: National Institutes of Health, 1990.

Corkin, S., Twitchell, T. E., et al. "Safety and Efficacy of Cingulotomy for Pain and Psychiatric Disorder." In Hitchcock, E. R., Ballantine, H. I. T., Myerson, B. A. (eds.), *Modern Concepts in Psychiatric Surgery.* New York: Elsevier/North Holland, 1979.

Crichton, Michael. *The Terminal Man.* New York: Alfred Knopf, 1972.

Delgado, José. *Physical Control of the Mind.* Volume 41 of the *World Perspective Series.* New York: Harper & Row, 1969.

Dodson, W. E., et al. "Management of Seizure Disorders: Selected Aspects, Parts I and II." *The Journal of Pediatrics,* vol. 89, 1976.

Flor-Henry, P. "Psychiatric Surgery, 1935–1973: Evaluation and Current Perspectives." *Journal of the Canadian Psychiatric Association,* vol. 20, 1975.

Ford, Mary Ellen. "A History of Lobotomy in the United States." *The Pharos,* 1987.

Fox, Peter. "Functional Brain Mapping with Position Emission Tomography." *Seminars in Neurology* 9(4), 1989.

Frank, Leonard R. "The Policies and Practices of American Psychiatry Are Oppressive." *Hospital and Community Psychiaty,* 1986.

Freeman, Walter. "Frontal Lobotomy in Early Schizophrenia: Long Follow-Up in 415 Cases." *British Journal of Psychiatry,* vol. 119, 1971.

Freeman, Walter. "Sexual Behavior and Fertility After Frontal Lobotomy." *Biological Psychiatry* 6(1), 1973.

Freeman, Walter, and Watts, James. *Psychosurgery in the Treatment of Mental Disorders and Intractable Pain.* Springfield: Charles C. Thomas, 1942.

Fulton, J. F. *Functional Localization on Relation to Frontal Lobotomy.* New York: Oxford University Press, 1949.

Fulton, J. F. *Frontal Lobotomy and Affective Behavior. A Neurophysiological Analysis.* London: Chapman and Hall, 1951.

Fulton, J. F., and Jacobsen, C. F. *The Functions of the Frontal Lobes: A Comparative Study in Monkeys, Chimpanzees and Man.* London: Abstracts of the Second International Neurological Congress, 1935.

Gaylin, Willard M. "The Problem of Psychosurgery." *Hastings Center Readings.*

Gazzaniga, Michael S., and Ledous, J. E. *The Integrated Mind.* New York: Plenum, 1978.

Gazzaniaga, Michael S. *The Social Brain.* New York: Basic Books, 1985.

Gazzaniga, Michael. *Mind Matters, How the Mind and Brain Interact to Create Our Conscious Lives.* Boston: Houghton Mifflin with MIT Press and Bradford Books, 1988.

Gazzaniga, Michael, "Organization of the Human Brain." *Science,* vol. 245, 1989.

Gelman, David. "Haunted by Their Habits." *Newsweek,* March 27, 1989.

Goffman, E. *Asylums: Essays on the Social Situation of Mental Patients and Other Inmates.* Garden City, NY: Doubleday Anchor, 1961.

Goldring, Sidney. "A Method for Surgical Management of Focal Epilepsy, Especially as It Related to Children." *Journal of Neurosurgery,* 1978.

Greenberg, Joel. "Altering Behavior with Brain Surgery." *The Boston Globe Magazine,* Jan. 1, 1978.

Gross, Martin. *The Psychological Society.* New York: Random House, 1978.

Hale, A. S., Bartlett, J. R., and Bridges, P. K. Lesion Size and Outcome Following the Psychosurgical Operation of Stereotactic Subcaudate Tractotomy. Submitted manuscript courtesy of authors, 1989.

Hale, Judson, *The Education of a Yankee: An American Memoir.* New York: Harper & Row, 1987.

Halleck, S. L. *Psychiatry and the Dilemmas of Crime: A Study of Causes, Punishment and Treatment.* New York: Harper & Hoeber, 1967.

Holden, J. M. C., et al. "Prefronatal Lobotomy, Stepping Stone or Pitfall." *American Journal of Psychiatry,* vol. 127, 1970.

Horsley, V., and Clarke, R. H. "The Structure and Functions of the Cerebellum Examined by a New Method." *Brain,* vol. 13, 1908.

Jenike, Michael, et al. Cingulotomy for Refractory Obsessive Compulsive Disorder: A Long-Term Follow-Up of 33 Patients. Manuscript courtesy of author.

Jenike, Michael, "Rapid Response of a Severe Obsessive Compulsive Neurosis to Tranylcypramine." *American Journal of Psychiatry,* vol. 138, 1981.

Kelly, D., Richardson, A., Mitchell-Heggs, N., Greenup, J., Chen, C., and Hafner, R. J. "Stereotactic Limbic Leukotomy. A Preliminary Report on 40 Patients." *British Journal of Psychiatry,* vol. 123, 1973.

Kesey, Ken. *One Flew Over the Cuckoo's Nest.* New York: S. French, 1970.

Kevles, Daniel J. *In the Name of Eugenics, Genetics and the Uses of Human Heredity.* New York: Alfred A. Knopf, 1985.

Kiloh, L. G., and Smith, J. S. "The Neural Basis of Aggression and Its Treatment by Psychosurgery." *Australian and New Zealand Journal of Psychiatry,* 1978.

Kiloh L. G. "Non-Pharmacological Biological Treatments of Psychiatry Patients." *Australian and New Zealand Journal of Psychiatry,* vol. 17, 1983.

Kluver, H., and Bucy P. C. "An Analysis of Certain Effects of Bilateral Temporal Lobectomy in the Rhesus Monkey with Special Reference to Psychic Blindness." *Journal of Psychology,* vol. 5, 1938.

Kluver, H., and Bucy P. C. "Psychic Blindness and Other Symptoms Following Bilateral Temporal Lobectomy in Rhesus Monkey." *American Journal of Physiology,* vol. 119, 1973.

Knight, G. "The Orbital Cortex as an Objective in the Surgical Treatment of Mental Illness. The Results of 450 Cases of Open Operation and the Development of the Stereotactic Approach." *British Journal of Surgery,* vol. 51, 1964.

Knight, G. C. "Intractable Psychoneurosis in the Elderly and Infirm, Treatment by Stereotactic Tractotomy." *British Journal of Geriatric Practice,* vol. 3, 1966.

Knight, G. C. "Stereotactic Surgery for the Relief of Suicidal and Severe Depression and Intractable Psychosneuroses." *Journal of Postgraduate Medicine,* vol. 45, 1969.

Knight, G. C. "Further Observations from an Experience of 660 Cases of Stereotactic Tractotomy." *Postgraduate Medical Journal,* vol. 49, 1973.

Knight, G. C. "Bifrontal Stereotactic Tractotomy: An Attraumatic Operations of Value in the Treatment of Intractable Psychoneurosis." *British Journal of Psychiatry,* vol. 115, 1969.

Knight, G. C. "Neurosurgical Aspects of Psychosurgery." *Proceedings of the Royal Society of Medicine,* vol. 65, 1972.

Knight, G. C., and Tredgold, R. F. "Orbital Leukotomy, A Review of 52 Cases." *Lancet,* 1955.

Kraepelin, E. *One Hundred Years of Psychiatry.* New York: Philosophical Library, 1962.

Kubos, Kenneth, Sanberg, Paul, and Moran, Timothy. "A Stereotaxic Positioning Platform for Double-Angle Placements." *Behavior Research Methods and Instrumentation* 15(1), 1983.

Kucharski, Anastasia. "History of Frontal Lobotomy in the United States, 1935–1955." *Neurosurgery,* vol. 14, 1984.

Lieberman, Jeffrey. "Evidence for a Biological Hypothesis of Obsessive Compulsive Disorder." *Neuropsychobiology,* vol. 11, 1984.

Livingston, K. E. "Cingulate Cortex Isolation for the Treatment of Psychoses and Psychoneuroses." *Association for Research of Nervous and Mental Disorders,* vol. 31, 1951.

Livingston, K. E. "Surgical Contributions to Psychiatric Treatment." In *American Handbook of Psychiatry,* vol. 5. New York: Basic Books, 1975.

Lovett, L. M., and Shaw, D. M. "Outcome in Bipolar Affective Disorders after Stereotactic Tractotomy." *Journal of British Psychiatry,* vol. 148, 1987.

Luria, A. R. *The Working Brain: An Introduction to Neuropsychology.* New York: Basic Books, 1973.

Mark, Vernon H. "A Psychosurgeon's Case for Psychosurgery." *Psychology Today,* 1974.

Mark, Vernon, and Ervin, Frank. *Violence and the Brain.* New York: Harper & Row, 1970.

Mark, V., Sweet, W., and Ervin, F. "Role of Brain Disease in Riots and Urban Violence." Letter. *Journal of the American Medical Association,* vol. 203, 1968.

Martuza, Robert, Chiocca, E. A., Jenike, Michael, Giriunas, I., and Ballantine, H. T. "Stereotactic Radiofrequency Thermal Cingulotomy for Obsessive Compulsive Disorder." *Journal of Neuropsychiatric Opinion* 2(3), Summer 1990.

Mason, B. "Brain Surgery to Control Behavior." *Ebony,* vol. 28, 1973.

Medhvedev, Zhores, and Medhvedev, Roy. *A Question of Madness.* New York: Alfred A. Knopf, 1971.

Miller, A. "The Lobotomy Patient—A Decade Later. A Follow-Up Study of a Research Project Started in 1948." *Journal of the Canadian Medical Association,* vol. 96, 1967.

Miller, Laurence. "The Emotional Brain." *Psychology Today,* 1988.

Mindus, P., Bergstrom, K., et al. "Magnetic Resonance Images Related to Clinical Outcome after Psychosurgical Intervention in Severe Anxiety Disorder." *Journal of Neurology, Neurosurgery, and Psychiatry,* vol. 50, 1987.

Mingrino, S., and Schergna, E. "Stereotactic Anterior Cingulotomy in the Treatment of Severe Behavior Disorders." In Hitchcock, E., et al. (eds.), *Psychosurgery.* Springfield, IL: Charles C. Thomas, 1972.

Moniz, Egas. "How I Succeeded in Performing the Prefrontal Lobotomy." In Sackler, A. M. *Great Physiodynamic Therapies in Psychiatry.* New York: Harper & Row, 1956.

Moser, Hanna M. "A Ten-Year Follow-Up of Lobotomy Patients." *Hospital and Community Psychiatry,* vol. 12, 1969.

Nauta, Haring. "A Simplified Perspective on the Basal Ganglia and Their Relation to the Limbic System." In Doane, B. K., and Livingston, K. E., (eds.), *The Limbic System: Functional Organization and Clinical Disorders.* New York: Raven Press, 1986.

Noonan, David. *Neuro—Life on the Frontlines of Brain Surgery and Neurological Medicine.* New York: Ivy Books, 1989.

Older, Jules. "Psychosurgery: Ethical Issues and a Proposal for Control." *American Journal of Orthopsychiatry,* 1974.

Papez, I. W. "A Proposed Mechanism of Emotion." *Archives of Neurology and Psychiatry,* vol. 38, 1937.

Pearlson, G. D., Veroff, A. E., and McHugh, P. R. "The Use of Computed Tomography in Psychiatry: Recent Application to Schizophrenia, Manic Depressive Illness and Dementia Syndrome." *Journal of Johns Hopkins Medicine,* 1981.

Perse, Teri. "Obsessive Compulsive Disorder: A Treatment Review." *Journal of Clinical Psychiatry,* vol. 49, 1988.

Petersen, S., Fox, P., Snyder, A., and Raichle, M. "Activation fo Extrastriate and Frontal Cortical Areas by Visual Words and Word-like Stimuli." *Science,* vol. 249, 1990.

Pisharodi, M., and Nauta, H. "An Animal Model for Neuron Specific Spinal Cord Lesions." Proceedings, 9th meeting World Society of Stereotactic and Functional Neurosurgery. Toronto. *Applied Neurophysiology,* vol. 48, 1985.

Poynton, A., Bridges, P., and Bartlett, J. "Psychosurgery in Britain Now." *British Journal of Neurosurgery,* 1988.

President's Commission for the Study of Ethical Problems in Medicine and Biomedical and Behavioral Research. *Protecting Human Subjects: The Adequacy and Uniformity of Federal Rules and Their Implementation.* Washington, DC: U.S. Government Printing Office, 1981.

Pressman, Jack D. "Sufficient Promise: John F. Fulton and the Origins of Psychosurgery." Richard H. Shryock Medal Essay, 1988.

"Psychosurgery." *Time*, November 30, 1942.

Raichle, Marcus, et al. "PET Studies in Panic Disorder." *Nature*, vol. 310, 1984.

Reiman, E. M., et al. "Neuroanatomical Correlates of a Lactate-Induced Anxiety Attack." *Archives of General Psychiatry*, vol. 46, 1989.

Reiman, E., Fusselman, J., Fox, P., and Raichel, M. "Neuroanatomical Correlates of Anticipatory Anxiety." *Science*, vol. 243, 1989.

Restak, Richard M. *The Brain*. New York: Bantam Books, 1984.

Rivers, Caryl. "Psychosurgery," unpublished manuscript, 1989.

Rodgers, J. "Psychiatry Suffers from Poor Image." *The News American*, May 7, 1978.

Scafr, Maggie. "Brain Researcher José Delgado Asks—What Kind of Humans Would We Like to Construct?" *New York Times Magazine*, November 15, 1970.

Schmidt, G., and Schorsch, E. "Psychosurgery of Sexually Deviant Patients: Review and Analysis of New Empirical Findings." *Archives of Sexual Behavior*, vol. 10, 1981.

Scoville, W. B. "Proposed Methods of Cortical Undercutting of Certain Areas of the Frontal Lobes as a Substitute for Prefrontal Lobotomy." *Digest of Neurology and Psychiatry*, vol. 16, 1948.

Scull, Andrew, and Favreau, Diane. "A Chance to Cut Is a Chance to Cure: Sexual Surgery for Psychosis in Three 19th-Century Societies." In *Research in Law, Deviance and Social Control*, vol. 8. JAI Press, 1986.

Shapiro, Michael H., and Spece, Roy G., Jr. *Bioethics and Law*. St. Paul: West Publishing, 1981.

Shevitz, Stewart. "Psychosurgery: Some Current Observations." *American Journal of Psychiatry*, vol. 133, 1976.

Shuman, Samuel I. *Psychosurgery and the Medical Control of Violence*. Detroit: Wayne State University Press, 1977.

Shutts, David. *Lobotomy, Resort to the Knife*. New York: Van Nostrand Reinhold, 1982.

Sigerist, Henry E. *A History of Medicine*. New York: Oxford University Press, 1951.

Snodgrass, Virginia. "Debate over Benefits and Ethics of Psychosurgery Involves the Public." *Journal of the American Medical Association*, 1973.

Snodgrass, Virginia. Psychosurgery Series. *Journal of the American Medical Association*, 1973.

Snyder, Solomon H. *Biological Aspects of Mental Disorder*. New York: Oxford University Press, 1980.

Standish-Barry. H. M. A. S., et al. "Pneumo-Encephalographic and Computerized Axial Tomography Scan Changes in Affective Disorders." *Journal of British Psychiatry*, 1982.

Strom-Olsen, R., and Carlisle, S. "Bifrontal Stereotactic Tractotomy." *British Journal of Psychiatry*, vol. 118, 1971.

Stuss, D. T., et al. "Language Functioning After Bilateral Prefrontal Leukotomy." *Brain and Language*, vol. 28, 1986.

Sugar, Oscar. "Changing Attitudes Toward Psychosurgery." *Journal of Surgical Neurology*, vol. 9, 1978.

Sweet, W. "Treatment of Medically Intractable Mental Disease by Limited Frontal Leukotomy—Justifiable?" *New England Journal of Medicine*, vol. 289, 1973.

Szasz, Thomas. *The Myth of Mental Illness*, New York: Harper & Hoeber, 1961.

Szasz, Thomas. *The Manufacture of Madness*. New York: Harper & Row, 1970.

Szasz, T. *The Age of Madness*. Garden City, NY: Anchor Doubleday, 1973.

Tetrud, James W., and Langston, J. W. "The Effect of Deprynl on the Natural History of Parkinson's Disease." *Science*, vol. 245, 1989

Tippin, J., and Henn, F. A. "Modified Leukotomy in the Treatment of Intractable Obsessional Neurosis." *American Journal of Psychiatry*, vol. 139, 1982.

Trotter, Robert. "Clockwork Orange in a California Prison." *Science News*, March 11, 1972.

Uematsu, S. "Surgical Management of Complex Partial Seizures." *JAMA*, vol. 264, 1990.

Uematsu, S., Rosenbaum, A., and Kumar, A. "Toward Computer Image-Controlled Electromechanical Stereotactic Brain Surgery." In Anderson, J. H. (ed.), *Medical Radiology Innovations in Diagnostic Radiology*. Berlin and Heidelberg: Springer-Verlag, 1989.

Urinous, Leroy F. "Brain Surgery Is Tested on Three California Convicts." *The Washington Post*, Feb. 25, 1972, A1.

Vaernet, K., and Madsen, A. "Stereotactic Amygdalotomy and Basofrontal Tractotomy in Psychotics with Aggressive Behavior." *Journal of Neurology, Neurosurgery, and Psychiatry*, vol. 33, 1970.

Valenstein, E. S. *Brain Control. A Critical Examination of Brain Stimulation and Psychosurgery.* John Wiley and Sons, 1973.

Valenstein, Elliot S. *Great and Desperate Cures. The Rise and Decline of Psychosurgery and Other Radical Treatments for Mental Illness.* New York: Basic Books, 1986.

Van Leeuwen, and Storm, W. "Intracerebral Interventions in Patients with Behavioral Disorders." *Journal of Psychiatry, Neurology, and Neurosurgery*, vol. 76, 1973.

Veatch, Robert M. "Generalization of Expertise." *Hastings Center Studies* 1(2), 1973.

Vinken, Pierre, Bruyn, George, and Klawans, Karold (eds.). *Handbook of Clinical Neurology.* Amsterdam: Elsevier Science Publishers, 1986.

Walker, Alan E., ed. *A History of Neurological Surgery,* 2nd ed. Hafner, 1967.

Weinberg, L. "Lobotomy: A Personal Memoir." *The Pharos,* 1988.

Winter, A. "Depression and Intractable Pain Treated by Modified Prefrontal Lobotomy." *Journal of the Medical Society of New Jersey* 69(9), 1972.

DATE DUE